DR. NEAL BARNARD'S
COOKBOOK
FOR
REVERSING
DIABETES

DR. NEAL BARNARD'S
COOKBOOK
— FOR —
REVERSING DIABETES

**150 RECIPES SCIENTIFICALLY PROVEN
TO REVERSE DIABETES WITHOUT DRUGS**

NEAL D. BARNARD, MD, FACC

WITH DREENA BURTON

RODALE

RODALE
wellness

Live happy. Be healthy. Get inspired.

Sign up today to get exclusive access to our authors, exclusive bonuses, and the most authoritative, useful, and cutting-edge information on health, wellness, fitness, and living your life to the fullest.

Visit us online at RodaleWellness.com
Join us at RodaleWellness.com/Join

Rodale books may be purchased for business or promotional use or for special sales. For information, please e-mail: BookMarketing@Rodale.com.

Printed in the United States of America

Rodale Inc. makes every effort to use acid-free ∞, recycled paper ♲.

Book design by Yeon Kim

Library of Congress Cataloging-in-Publication Data is on file with the publisher.

ISBN 978–1–62336–929–3

Distributed to the trade by Macmillan

2 4 6 8 10 9 7 5 3 1 hardcover

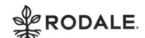

We inspire health, healing, happiness, and love in the world.

Starting with you.

This book is dedicated to our research participants,
to the team at the Physicians Committee for Responsible Medicine,
and to our many friends and colleagues who have
brought forward new power to tackle diabetes.

CONTENTS

A NOTE TO THE READER

The program you are about to begin takes a powerful approach to diabetes. Our focus is not on pills or shots, but on foods, and it is the most delicious "prescription" you could imagine. A dietary change can dramatically improve your health and can sometimes even make diabetes go away, for all intents and purposes.

Before we begin, let me share some important tips.

SEE YOUR DOCTOR • Let your doctor know that you are improving your eating habits. It's not that dietary changes are dangerous. Quite the opposite—they are extraordinarily healthful. But the combination of a powerful change in your diet, along with medications you may already be taking, can mean that your blood sugar could actually fall too low. And exercise can drop your blood sugar even further. So be sure to speak with your doctor before you start, so that your medications can be adjusted or stopped when the time is right.

USE A BLOOD GLUCOSE METER • Your meter will help you track your progress and help you to know if your blood sugar is dipping low enough that your doctor should reduce or stop your medications.

GET COMPLETE NUTRITION • Although the foods you'll learn about in this book are very nutritious—more so than those recommended in other diabetes regimens—there are two supplements that I highly recommend.

- Vitamin B_{12} is essential for healthy nerves and healthy blood cells, but it is not made by plants or animals. So as you begin a plant-based diet, it is important to take a B_{12} supplement. That can mean a typical daily multiple vitamin—all of which contain B_{12}—or a stand-alone vitamin B_{12} supplement. All drugstores and health food stores carry B_{12} supplements that meet or exceed the recommended daily allowance. We will talk more about vitamin B_{12} in Chapter 3.

● Vitamin D helps your body absorb calcium from the foods you eat and also helps prevent cancer. In sunny locales, sunlight on your skin can produce all the vitamin D you need. However, if you live in a not-so-sunny spot, stay indoors for much of the time, or use sunscreen, you are likely to be low in vitamin D. A supplement of 2,000 IU per day is safe and helpful.

SHARE THIS INFORMATION • You may know other people who are dealing with diabetes, excess weight, or other health issues. Many have not heard of the approach that is in your hands now, and they will benefit enormously if you will share what you have learned with them.

Now, let's jump in!

INTRODUCTION

At Yale University, researchers turned our understanding of type 2 diabetes on its head. At the time, a common belief was that diabetes was caused by eating too much sugar or too many carbohydrate-rich foods, such as bread or potatoes. That was an understandable notion, because people with diabetes have too much sugar in their bloodstreams. It made sense to think that maybe the whole problem was that they had too much candy, soda, bread, etc., in their diets. Hundreds of guides were written advising people to limit sugar, potatoes, fruit, pasta, beans, and other sweet or starchy foods. Unfortunately, these dietary changes didn't help very much.

But using a high-tech scanning technology called magnetic resonance spectroscopy, the Yale researchers looked inside the cells of people with diabetes, and what they found revolutionized our understanding of this disease.

Hidden inside muscle and liver cells, the Yale team found microscopic particles of fat. This was not belly fat or thigh fat; it was fat *inside* the muscle and liver cells. It had come from the foods the research participants had been eating, and it had lodged in their cells. Once inside, those fat particles kept sugar from entering the cells. More specifically, the fat particles interfered with insulin—the hormone that normally escorts sugar into cells. If insulin can no longer move sugar into cells, sugar builds up outside your cells, in your bloodstream.

In other words, diabetes isn't caused by eating too much sugar or carbohydrate. Rather, it apparently starts with fat building up inside the cells. And that causes *insulin resistance*—insulin no longer works normally. And it also became clear that the answer to type 2 diabetes is not to avoid potatoes, bread, fruit, or other sweet or starchy foods, but rather to counteract the fat buildup inside the cells.

At the Physicians Committee for Responsible Medicine, our research team has been working on ways to do just that. We tested a diet that had no animal fat at all and very little vegetable oil. In theory, this ought to cause that intracellular fat buildup to start to disappear. In a head-to-head test, we compared this low-fat vegan diet with a conventional "diabetes diet" in people with type 2 diabetes.

The results were spectacular. After 22 weeks, the vegan diet led to a threefold greater improvement in blood sugar control, compared with the conventional diabetes diet. This was all the more remarkable because the people on the conventional diet were carefully limiting their portions and trying not to overdo it on carbs, while the vegan group participants were free to eat as much food as they wished, with no limits on calories, carbohydrates, or portion sizes, and they made no changes to their exercise patterns or medications. The dietary change alone slashed their blood sugar levels. They also improved their cholesterol levels and lost weight. It turned out to be an extraordinarily powerful dietary approach to diabetes and all the health problems that go with it.

If this wonderful news is something you have not heard before—or if your doctor never mentioned any of this—the reason is that our National Institutes of Health study findings were first published by the American Diabetes Association in *Diabetes Care* in 2006, and some doctors are still treating diabetes based on the knowledge they picked up before that date. Moreover, in medical training, pharmaceuticals have eclipsed nutrition—even for conditions like diabetes or high cholesterol levels, where food choices are the central consideration. Doctors have focused their attention on drugs, even though food changes are often safer, more powerful, and much more patient-friendly.

HOW DOES IT TASTE?

How did the participants feel about this way of eating? After all, they were not eating meat, cheese, or any other animal products, and greasy french fries and oily foods were out, too. Did they like the food, or did they feel deprived?

To answer that question, we asked our participants about their dietary changes in great detail. And they told us that this new approach was life-changing. Not only was it powerful; many were also surprised to find that it was easier than other diets—much easier than limiting calories or counting carbohydrate grams, and a great relief from the low-carb diets that made them feel guilty for wanting a slice of bread or a baked potato.

Because they were free to eat as much as they wanted, they were never hungry. And the wide range of dishes and delicious flavors included in the plan meant that they were really enjoying eating, as opposed to resigning themselves to the bland diets many had been on before. They tried new flavors, new recipes, new food products, and new restaurant choices. For many, the experience was less like a diet and more like an adventure. Take a look at the recipes in this book, and you'll see what I mean. There are wonderful tastes waiting for you.

Most importantly, our participants were rewarded. Unwanted weight disappeared without exercise. Their need for medications fell day by day. Many reported having more energy than they had had in years. Their laboratory tests looked better and better. And they felt power and a sense of control over their diabetes that they had never felt before.

So if you would like to lose weight, tackle diabetes, or improve other health conditions, you have come to the right place. Culinary traditions from all around the world have explored plant-based foods for millennia, and now it's your turn. The recipes in this book are as delightful to your taste buds as they are powerful for your health. Some recipes put a healthy twist on old favorites, and others let you explore some new flavors.

As you begin, I'd like to invite you to take advantage of other helpful resources. If you have not yet read *Dr. Neal Barnard's Program for Reversing Diabetes,* I encourage you to take advantage of the detailed information it holds. My other books tackle additional important health topics, from preventing Alzheimer's disease to stopping chronic pain. And my organization, the Physicians Committee for Responsible Medicine, has a number of innovative programs and opportunities that you can learn about on its Web site, PCRM.org. These include:

- The 21-Day Vegan Kickstart, a free online program providing daily recipes, menus, and cooking videos, starting fresh every month.
- The Food for Life program, which is taught by trained instructors and provides nutrition and cooking classes in dozens of communities.
- Our continuing education program for physicians, nurses, dietitians, and other health-care professionals, as well as our annual International Conference on Nutrition in Medicine.
- The Barnard Medical Center, which provides complete nutrition evaluations and guidance as an integral part of medical care.

Dreena Burton, who provided the wonderful recipes in this book, has a number of excellent books, too, and runs Dreena Burton's Plant-Powered Kitchen (dreenaburton.com).

I hope you enjoy this exploration and learn many new things that you can share with others. I wish you the very best of health!

PREFACE

WHAT DOES IT MEAN TO REVERSE DIABETES?

In 2003, a man came to our research center at the Physicians Committee for Responsible Medicine to join a study on type 2 diabetes. His family had suffered enormously from the disease, and he had been diagnosed at the age of 31. When he began the study, his blood sugar was elevated, and he had a great deal of weight to lose. But as he began to follow a low-fat, plant-based diet under our direction, everything changed. Excess weight melted away, and his blood sugar came down. And down. And down. As the weeks went by, his personal physician was impressed by his progress and stopped his diabetes medication. He just did not need it anymore. Eventually, his blood tests improved to the point that there was no trace of diabetes left. He was on no diabetes medications at all, and his blood sugar was squarely in the normal range.

This raised a question: What should we tell him? I had been taught—as you may have been, too—that diabetes never goes away. "Once you have diabetes, you'll always have diabetes," was what people said. And yet here was a man who had had diabetes for years, but who was now on no medication and who had perfectly normal blood sugar. He could walk into any medical clinic in the world and no one would have guessed that he had ever had the disease. Should we tell him that his diabetes was gone?

As time went on, that question became easier to answer, thanks to our surgical friends. Patients who lose hundreds of pounds after bariatric surgery often find their diabetes disappearing, so doctors have become more comfortable with the notion of type 2 diabetes being a two-way street. Many have found that, when people lose a great deal of weight or make big changes to their diets, the blood tests can, in some cases, show a return to the normal range.

However "reversing" is not a medical term. When I speak of "reversing type 2 diabetes," what I mean is that the disease process turns around. Weight that has been steadily rising starts moving in the opposite direction. Cholesterol and blood pressure numbers that have been steadily going up begin falling. Blood sugar values that have been hard to control finally begin to drop, too—often to the point where medications must be reduced or stopped. Sometimes type 2 diabetes improves so much that it is simply no longer detectable. And complications, such as painful neuropathy, can release their grip, too.

Remember: Type 1 diabetes is different. It requires continued insulin treatments, regardless of how well you adjust your diet. Nonetheless, diet changes are very helpful for type 1 diabetes, too, as we will see shortly.

For any individual, it is not possible to know in advance how much your diabetes will improve. So the thing to do is to get started. I wish you every success with this powerful program!

CHAPTER 1

TURNING DIABETES AROUND

LET'S take a quick look at a couple of basics: what diabetes means and why a diet change can be so powerful.

Diabetes means there is too much sugar in your blood. That sugar—called *glucose*—powers your body. At least, that is what it is supposed to do. Glucose provides energy to allow your muscles to move, your brain to think, and all the rest of you to do the things your body is designed for. In the same way that a car runs on gasoline, your cells run on glucose.

When you have diabetes, glucose has trouble moving into your cells, where it belongs. Instead, it builds up in your bloodstream. The problem is insulin, a hormone made in your pancreas. Insulin normally acts like a key, opening up a cell's outer membrane to let glucose inside. In diabetes, insulin is falling down on the job. It is not getting glucose into your cells very well, so your body does not have the energy source it needs. You'll feel run-down and tired. Worse, the glucose building up in your bloodstream circulates through the delicate blood vessels of your heart, eyes, kidneys, and other organs and can damage them.

So if gasoline can't get into your gas tank, your car can't move. And if gasoline spills all over your garage floor, it can be corrosive. You need gas in your tank and glucose in your cells. If gas and glucose don't go where they belong, things don't work right.

THREE MAIN TYPES

There are three main types of diabetes—type 1, type 2, and gestational.

TYPE 1 DIABETES used to be called *childhood-onset* or *insulin-dependent* diabetes. In this form of the disease, the insulin-producing cells have been destroyed by an autoimmune reaction. That is, antibodies in the bloodstream have attacked the pancreas, killing the beta cells that make insulin.

TYPE 2 DIABETES is much more common than type 1. This condition was once called *adult-onset* or *non-insulin-dependent* diabetes. However, in countries where meaty, dairy-heavy diets lead to obesity and to the buildup of fat particles inside muscle and liver cells, type 2 diabetes is found in many adolescents.

In this form of diabetes, the pancreas is still making insulin, but the cells do not respond to it normally, as discussed above. To try to overcome insulin resistance, the pancreas makes more and more insulin to force glucose into the cells. But eventually, the pancreas loses some of its insulin-making ability, and blood sugar levels rise.

GESTATIONAL DIABETES is similar to type 2, but it occurs during pregnancy. Although it disappears when pregnancy is over, it is a sign that type 2 diabetes could soon arise. Like type 2, it relates to insulin resistance, and the same dietary improvements that help prevent type 2 can help prevent gestational diabetes.

FOODS AND TYPE 2 DIABETES

Type 2 diabetes is common among meat-eaters. But it is much less common among people who avoid meat and is rare among people who avoid animal products altogether. As I mentioned in the Introduction, our research team at the Physicians Committee for Responsible Medicine has pioneered the exploration of dietary approaches to type 2 diabetes. In the 1990s, we tested a low-fat vegan diet—that is, a diet without animal products—in a small pilot study, working with our colleagues at Georgetown University. The study was short—just 12 weeks—and we had only 13 participants. Even so, the results were dramatic, prompting our team and others to launch several new studies to test this powerful new dietary approach. Of these, the best known was our NIH trial, the results of which were published by the American Diabetes Association in 2006 in *Diabetes Care.* In that study, the improvement in A1C—the blood test commonly used to track blood sugar control—was three times greater on the vegan diet than on a conventional diabetes diet in people who made no changes to their medications or exercise patterns. In fact, the improvement in A1C was greater than is seen with oral diabetes medications. Follow-up results were published by the *American Journal of Clinical Nutrition,* the *Journal of the American Dietetic Association,* and other publications.

We later worked with people with *diabetic neuropathy*—a condition that causes pain and sometimes numbness during later-stage diabetes. We found that a low-fat vegan diet not only improves blood sugar and overall health, but it also reduces and sometimes eliminates painful symptoms and improves nerve function.

WHAT ABOUT TYPE 1?

For people with type 1 diabetes, a dietary change is important, too. It will not eliminate the need for insulin, but it can provide two very important benefits.

First, it can reduce the amount of insulin you require. For reasons that are not entirely clear, people with type 1 diabetes who begin a low-fat vegan diet often find that their blood sugars are well-controlled with less insulin than they were using before.

Second, a dietary change can help prevent complications. Diabetes attacks the blood vessels to the heart, eyes, kidneys, and extremities, and the damage to blood vessels in the brain may help explain why diabetes doubles your risk of Alzheimer's disease. If you have type 1 diabetes, protecting your blood vessels is critical, so you do not want *any* animal fat or cholesterol in your diet. A plant-based diet is the best eating style for controlling your weight, blood sugar, cholesterol, and blood pressure, all of which are important for maintaining the health of your arteries.

In addition to *managing* type 1 diabetes, food also appears to play a key role in *preventing* it. In 1992, researchers from Canada and Finland revealed some groundbreaking findings. They had taken blood samples from 142 children with type 1 diabetes and had found that every single child had antibodies to cow's milk proteins. Normally, your body makes antibodies to act as little torpedoes to destroy invading viruses, bacteria, or cancer cells. But in these children, antibodies had formed against the proteins in milk. In turn, it appeared that the antibodies to cow's milk had also attacked the children's own pancreatic cells, leading to diabetes. At least that is what the evidence suggested, and other researchers have been looking at whether avoiding cow's milk can help prevent the disease.

The obvious first step is to breastfeed children. The second is to avoid animal milk products. This makes sense not just for the child, but also for a breastfeeding mother, because dairy proteins she ingests as milk or cheese, for example, can end up in her breast milk and reach her baby.

This book puts this science to work. All of the recipes are free of animal products and emphasize healthful ingredients. You won't find a scrap of animal fat or cholesterol, and you'll have zero exposure to cow's milk proteins and whatever reactions they might cause.

HOW FOODS PROTECT YOUR HEALTH

Let's take a minute to see how plant-based foods work their magic.

THEY TACKLE YOUR BLOOD SUGAR • As we've seen, a plant-based eating pattern is far more effective than a typical "diabetes diet." The type 2 diabetes diets that are commonly prescribed at many medical clinics are far behind the times. First, old-fashioned diets try to make you starve off excess pounds by cutting calories—typically 500 a day. So if you normally eat 1,800 calories per day, your new diet will allow you only 1,300. For most people, that gets old fast; they feel hungry and drained. Second, conventional diets ask you to limit carbohydrates and keep your carbohydrate intake steady from meal to meal and from day to day. The idea is, if your carbohydrate intake stays steady, it is easier to pick the right dose of glucose-lowering medications. In other words, you are now simply eating for your medications. These conventional diets were devised before we knew what we now do about what causes diabetes.

A plant-based diet is dramatically different. It targets the *cause* of type 2 diabetes. It aims to reverse the fat buildup inside your cells, tackle your insulin resistance, and bring your blood sugar down decisively. It does not cater to your medications; the goal is to reduce or eliminate them to the extent possible.

THEY HELP YOU LOSE WEIGHT • People who follow plant-based diets are slimmer, on average, than people following other diets. For many years, researchers have studied large groups of people, tracking their diets and weighing them. Seventh-day Adventists have been under special scrutiny because, as a group, they are particularly health conscious, avoiding tobacco and alcohol and, in many cases, adopting a vegetarian diet. In studies of Adventists, an average person following a vegan diet weighed 35 pounds less than his or her meat-eating friends! In fact, when comparing meat-eaters, semi-vegetarians, pescatarians, lacto-ovo vegetarians, and vegans, people following a vegan diet were the *only* group whose average weight was squarely in the healthy range. Studies have also shown that when people begin a low-fat vegan diet, excess weight tends to fall away.

So how does this happen? Why does a plant-based diet cause the pounds to melt away? For starters, fruits, vegetables, beans, and grains are rich in complex carbohydrates and contain very little fat. Cheese and meat are the opposite: They're high in fat and devoid of carbohydrates. Here is why this matters: Fat packs nine calories into every gram, while carbohydrate contains only four calories per gram. In other words, animal products are often loaded with calories, while plant products are not.

Also, these same fruits, vegetables, beans, and whole grains are rich in fiber, and fiber fills you up but contains essentially no calories. You tend to push away from the table before you've overeaten. But meat is not a plant, so it has no fiber. The same goes for dairy products and eggs. Fiber is found only in plants. So when you eat cheese, meat, or other animal products, you get every last calorie they hold, with no fiber to protect you from overeating. But plant-based foods are loaded with appetite-taming fiber.

Finally, our research has shown that when people begin a low-fat, plant-based diet, their after-meal metabolisms increase slightly. That means that you are burning calories faster for a few hours after breakfast, lunch, and dinner.

So we can see why a low-fat, plant-based diet helps you trim down and also helps you avoid future weight gain. As delicious as these foods are, they are modest in calories, there is plenty of fiber to tame your appetite, and they give a little boost to your after-meal calorie-burning speed.

THEY TRIM YOUR CHOLESTEROL • Meats and other animal-based foods contain cholesterol. So when you eat them, some of that cholesterol passes into your bloodstream, adding to whatever cholesterol was already there. This can contribute to artery blockages that can damage your heart. Worse, dairy products, meat, and eggs contain *saturated fat,* which causes your cholesterol levels to rise, and the effect of saturated fat is greater than the effect of the cholesterol in these foods.

Foods from plant sources are completely different. They have essentially no cholesterol and very little saturated fat. Many are rich in *soluble fiber,* which actually helps your body eliminate cholesterol.

THEY HELP LOWER YOUR BLOOD PRESSURE • When people adopt a plant-based diet, their blood pressure tends to fall. Scientists attribute this to several factors. First, plants are rich in potassium, which lowers blood pressure. Second, because vegetables, fruits, and other plant-based foods are low in "bad" fats, they tend to make your blood less thick, or less *viscous,* than animal products do. Third, as a plant-based diet trims away unwanted weight, your blood pressure is likely to fall further.In the next chapter, we will show you how to turn these powerful scientific findings into delicious foods.

CHAPTER 2

PACKING POWER INTO EVERY MEAL

METFORMIN, the most common medication prescribed to patients with type 2 diabetes, is not especially tasty. Let it sit on your tongue for a while, and you'll see what I mean. And its most common side effect is digestive upset. It does reduce your blood sugar a bit, and some people certainly do benefit from metformin and other diabetes medications. I don't mean to suggest that you shouldn't use them. But the foods you are about to try taste a whole lot better, and their combined effect is much greater than any effect oral medications could ever hope to have. And when it comes to healthful, plant-based foods, their side effects are ones you actually want: a slimmer waistline, more energy, and better health.

A diet for turning diabetes around should do three things: set animal products aside, keep vegetable oils to a minimum, and favor low–Glycemic Index (GI) foods. Let me show you how this works. Along the way, you'll notice what we are *not* doing: We are not setting any limit on calories, and we are not avoiding carbohydrates. Instead of focusing on *how much* you eat, we will focus on *what* you eat. The idea is to eat until you are satisfied and to be sure that the foods on your plate are healthful.

Here are the three keys to this diet.

1. **SET ANIMAL PRODUCTS ASIDE** • We are going to skip meat, poultry, fish, dairy products, and eggs. That means there will be no animal fat on your plate at all, and no cholesterol. Because everything you eat comes from plant sources, your foods will be loaded with fiber and vitamins, which is a great advantage for your health.

    "What, no fish?" you might be asking. That's right. Fish is much more like beef than it is like broccoli. It has no complex carbohydrates and no fiber, but it does contribute fat and cholesterol to your diet. In fact, some people choose fish precisely *because* it is fatty. They are piling on the salmon, imagining that its omega-3 fats will work some sort of biological magic. And salmon really is loaded with fat. Atlantic salmon is about 40 percent fat, as a percentage of calories. Chinook salmon is more than 50 percent fat. That is a lot. And while some of that fat is indeed omega-3, most of it is not. Salmon and other fish contribute a load of saturated fat, and, like any other fats, fish fats are dense in calories—which is why salmon lovers often have trouble with their weight. As a group, they are significantly heavier and have a higher risk of developing diabetes than people following plant-based diets.

    If you are wondering how you'll get enough calcium on a dairy-free diet, you'll find plenty in green leafy vegetables and beans. (More on this in the next chapter.)

2. **KEEP VEGETABLE OILS TO A MINIMUM** • Although vegetable oils are much more healthful than animal fats—they are typically much lower in *saturated fat*—they are still high in calories, and it pays to keep them to a minimum. That means using fat-free food preparation methods.

3. **FAVOR LOW-GLYCEMIC INDEX FOODS** • The Glycemic Index (GI) is a guide to how foods affect your blood sugar. For example, white bread tends to make blood sugar rise significantly. Rye bread is gentler on your blood sugar, and pumpernickel even more so. So white bread has a high GI, while pumpernickel has a lower GI.

Researchers have tested the GIs of hundreds and hundreds of foods. But let's simplify things. Here is all you really need to know.

- Instead of processed foods containing sugar, have fruit. Yes, fruit is sweet, but it has much less effect on your blood sugar.
- Instead of wheat breads, choose rye or pumpernickel.
- Instead of white potatoes, have sweet potatoes.
- Instead of typical cold cereals, eat oatmeal or bran cereal.

Beans and green vegetables are GI stars, having very little effect on your blood sugar. And surprisingly, pasta (even white pasta) has a low GI because, unlike bread, which is light and fluffy thanks to the yeast used in the baking process, pasta is more dense and compact, so its natural sugars are released only very slowly.

FOUR HEALTHFUL FOOD GROUPS

So now that you know what you want to eliminate from your diet, it's time to talk about what to include. As you build your meals, you'll start with four healthful food groups: vegetables, fruits, whole grains, and legumes (beans, peas, and lentils). Think of them as the palette from which your meals will be created.

VEGETABLES • There is an endless variety of vegetables. You want to get to know *cruciferous* vegetables, so named for their cross-shaped flowers. This group includes broccoli, cauliflower, kale, collards, Brussels sprouts, and many others. They are rich in highly absorbable calcium and have been shown to help prevent cancer.

You'll also want to eat plenty of orange vegetables, such as carrots and sweet potatoes. They get their color from beta-carotene, a powerful antioxidant.

Although many people treat vegetables as an afterthought, our meals put them front and center. And why not have two or more vegetables at a meal, such as broccoli and carrots, or sweet potatoes and asparagus?

FRUITS • Fruits are the original fast foods. They are loaded with vitamins and antioxidants and are great as snacks, desserts, or full meals, if you like. You are already familiar with apples, bananas, oranges, peaches, pears, and other grocery store staples. But branch out and try tropical papayas and mangoes, if you have not already, as well as berries, including blueberries, raspberries, etc.

Despite their sweet taste, most fruits have a low Glycemic Index. Although watermelon and pineapple have somewhat higher GIs, they are mostly water, so there is really not a great deal of sugar in them, and I suggest enjoying them just like you would other fruits.

As you select your vegetables and fruits, look for color. Orange, red, and purple—these colors mean antioxidants. (Orange means beta-carotene, red means lycopene, and purple means anthocyanins, to be specific.) And green leafy vegetables are typically rich in iron and calcium.

WHOLE GRAINS • Rice, oats, barley, and dozens of other grains—and the delicious foods made from them—are loaded with healthful complex carbohydrates and fiber. Whole grains have health advantages that refined grains don't. When a grain's outer bran coating is removed, it loses its fiber, as, for example, when brown rice is converted to white rice or when whole wheat is converted to white flour.

Even so, when researchers have tested white pasta, they've found its GI to be remarkably healthy, as I mentioned earlier—even though it has very little fiber. The reason, again, is that pasta is highly compacted and digests slowly, so it has less effect on blood sugar than white bread, which has air pockets and therefore releases its sugars more quickly than pasta does.

Some people are going gluten-free. Gluten is a protein found in wheat, barley, and rye. About 1 percent of the population has celiac disease (a sensitivity to the gluten protein), so they really do need to avoid these grains. Some other people—perhaps 1 in 10—feel better when they avoid gluten, too. Their digestion is better and they feel better mentally. But most people can eat wheat, barley, and rye with no problem.

LEGUMES • "Legumes" is a fancy word for beans, peas, and lentils. Pinto beans, black beans, chickpeas, navy beans, soybeans—these simple foods were staples for our grandparents but have been forgotten in recent years. You'll want to bring them into your life. They give you protein without cholesterol, calcium without saturated fat, and plenty of soluble fiber, and they boast a remarkably low Glycemic Index.

Try lentil or split pea soup as a savory start to a meal. Pinto or black beans can fill a burrito or taco, and chickpeas can top a salad or turn into hummus to spread on a sandwich or use as a dip. Soybeans have been turned into everything from soy milk and tofu to yogurt, cheese, bacon, and sausage. All of these soy alternatives are far healthier than the products they replace.

By the way, if you have bought into the "soy is unhealthy" myth, let me say a quick word to try to make sense of it for you. A century ago, researchers discovered compounds in soybeans and many other foods called *isoflavones*. Because their chemical structure looked vaguely like testosterone, estrogen, and other hormones, some reasoned that isoflavones might act like hormones, impairing fertility and promoting cancer.

The opposite is actually true: Soy products have no harmful effect on fertility at all. And a 2014 meta-analysis summarizing the results of 35 prior studies showed that women who consume the most soy products (soy milk, tofu, etc.) have about a 40 percent *lower* risk of developing breast cancer, compared with their soy-avoiding friends. Similarly, in a report based on the experiences of 9,514 women who had been previously treated for breast cancer, those who consumed the most soy had about a 30 percent reduction in their risk that the cancer would return, compared with women who generally avoided soy products. Among men, soy products appear to reduce the risk of prostate cancer.

Soy products are not essential for good health, but they are handy, and evidence suggests that they may help prevent cancer. As we saw above, women who include soy milk, tofu, and other soy products in their diets are less likely to develop breast cancer. If they had previously been treated for breast cancer, these same foods are also associated with better odds for survival.

FROM INGREDIENTS TO MEALS

Vegetables, fruits, grains, and legumes are ingredients. On your plate, they translate into angel hair pasta topped with artichoke hearts and seared oyster mushrooms, a chunky vegetable chili, butternut squash soup, Cuban black beans and rice, and many other possibilities.

Page through the recipes starting on page 24. You'll find a Caesar dressing that is lusciously creamy but that doesn't contain a drop of dairy or oil, as well as the most delicious chili you've ever tasted. No one has to know that cauliflower and carrots are hidden inside. How about a burger and onion rings? We'll show you how to make them in a healthful way, without a speck of meat or dairy products. Or savor our Cocoa Carrot Muffins (page 44) or our Strawberry Chia Pudding (page 196). Even as your taste buds are rejoicing, your body is regaining its health.

FOR EXTRA CREDIT

Two more bits of advice:

- Incorporate raw foods into your diet. For some reason, raw foods seem to add extra weight-loss power. Most fruits are great raw, and many vegetables are, as well. (By the way, this is *not* true of broccoli and other cruciferous vegetables, which need to be cooked to be digestible.)

- Also, do not avoid carbs. Some chronic dieters have trouble freeing themselves of the "carbs are fattening" myth. But when you cross rice, pasta, and sweet potatoes off your shopping list, you are missing out on the foods that have kept populations thin and healthy over millennia— and condemning yourself to a lifetime of weight struggles. Take an orange crayon and write on your refrigerator door, "Carbs have only four calories per gram; fats have nine!" And enjoy healthful, carbohydrate-rich foods. These foods are modest in calories and will help you stay slim.

In the next chapter, we will look at getting complete nutrition. It's easy. And be sure to pay careful attention to the section on vitamin B_{12}.

CHAPTER 3

COMPLETE NUTRITION

A MENU of vegetables, fruits, whole grains, and legumes gives your body the nutrition it needs but requires remarkably little menu planning. In this chapter, we will look at how to make sure you are not missing anything. As you will see, getting the nutrition you need is very easy. In fact, much of this chapter aims to convince you *not* to worry about nutrients that need little, if any, attention.

Even so, there are a few things that merit some discussion—I'm thinking especially of vitamin B_{12} and vitamin D—so let's start there.

VITAMIN B_{12} • You need B_{12} for healthy nerves and healthy blood cells. But B_{12} is not made by either plants or animals; it is made by bacteria. Some people have speculated that, before the advent of modern hygiene, the bacteria in soil, on plants, on our fingers, or in our mouths gave us the B_{12} traces we need. Whether that was ever true is hard to say, but it is certainly not true today.

Meat-eaters get some B_{12} because the bacteria in a cow's gut make it, and traces pass into meat and milk. We have similar bacteria in our digestive tracts, but scientists believe that it is produced too far down in our intestines to be absorbed.

A great many people have trouble absorbing B_{12} from animal products. That's because B_{12} is bound to proteins. If you are not producing much stomach acid—perhaps because you are taking an acid-blocking medication or are simply not making as much stomach acid as you used to—you may not be absorbing B_{12} very well. Also, metformin reduces B_{12} absorption, and because metformin is the most commonly prescribed medicine for type 2 diabetes, you can see why people—especially those with diabetes—might run low.

The answer is a supplement. Unlike the vitamin B_{12} found in animal products, the B_{12} in supplements is easily absorbed. The recommended dietary allowance of B_{12} is tiny—just 2.4 micrograms per day for adults—and all common multivitamins include more than that. Drugstores and health-food stores also stock supplements containing B_{12} alone, as well as supplements combining B_{12} with other B vitamins. They are all fine. There are no risks associated with taking too much B_{12}—the vitamin is safe even if taken in large amounts.

Some foods—including breakfast cereals, soy milk, and nutritional yeast—are fortified with the vitamin, too. But to be sure you are getting the amount you need, it's a good idea to take a supplement regularly.

VITAMIN D • As we discussed earlier, vitamin D helps your body absorb calcium and helps protect you from cancer, as well as performing other functions. Your body normally produces vitamin D when your skin is exposed to sunlight. When our forebears lived in equatorial Africa, the plentiful sunshine gave them all the vitamin D they needed. But somewhere along the line, our restless ancestors moved to places like North Dakota, Seoul, and Oslo, and sunlight was less plentiful. Moreover, if you are indoors most of the day or you use sunscreen, you are not getting your normal dose of sunlight. So it makes sense to take a supplement. A dose of up to 2,000 international units (IU) per day appears to be safe.

If you are unsure if you really need a supplement, your doctor can check your vitamin D level. If you are not getting regular sun exposure, however, it is safe to assume that you need a vitamin D supplement.

So vitamin B_{12} and vitamin D are the two vitamins worth thinking about. A B_{12} supplement is mandatory and a vitamin D supplement is a good idea.

Let's have a look at protein, calcium, and iron. These are dietary needs that are often discussed but are really very simple to get.

PROTEIN • Protein is used to repair body tissues and to make various molecules that your body uses. But here is the key: The amount you need is surprisingly modest. Although protein is often a preoccupation of people who are considering a dietary change, most people get far more than they need.

You'll find plenty of protein in beans, grains, and vegetables. Broccoli, spinach, and other greens are about one-third protein or even more, as a percentage of calories. If that sounds surprising, picture a bull, stallion, elephant, or giraffe. All of them build their massive bodies entirely from plant-based foods.

Here are a few more details: You probably know that proteins are built from amino acids. Like beads in a necklace, the amino acids link together to form protein strands. Your body can make some of these amino acids, while others (called *essential amino acids*) cannot be made in your body and have to come from foods. The good news is that all of the essential amino acids—all of the protein building blocks you need—are found in plants. There is no need to carefully combine specific food groups in search of this or that amino acid. Any normal varied diet built from vegetables, fruits, beans, and grains will provide all of the amino acids you need.

This is also true for athletes. Yes, they need more protein than sedentary people do to repair the wear and tear on their bodies. But a plant-based diet still provides more than enough protein, even for the most vigorous athlete.

Bottom line: On any normal, varied, plant-based diet, you'll get the protein you need without thinking about it. Just as breathing gives you oxygen without your having to measure it, eating foods from plants gives you all the protein you need.

CALCIUM • Your body needs calcium for bone development and many other things. But you do not need dairy calcium. After all, only about 30 percent of the calcium in milk is absorbed by your body. And along with it come lactose (a type of sugar), dairy fats, hormones, and other things you *don't* want.

There is plenty of highly absorbable calcium in green leafy vegetables. Broccoli, kale, collards, Brussels sprouts, and other greens are loaded with it. Think about it: A cow doesn't make the calcium found in its milk. A cow simply ingests the calcium in green leafy vegetables—that is, grass. You can do the same, albeit with a tastier selection of greens! Green vegetables are nature's best calcium source. An exception to this rule is spinach: Unlike other greens, the calcium in spinach is not well absorbed.

Calcium is also found in many other foods, particularly beans. So when it comes to calcium, think "greens and beans."

IRON • Greens and beans provide iron, too. You already know that you need iron to build hemoglobin, which allows your red blood cells to transport oxygen, and these healthful plant foods provide plenty of it. If you are eating red meat for the iron it contains, keep in mind that cows do not make iron. Cows get iron from the same source as they do calcium—from grass and other plant foods.

It is actually better to get iron directly from plant sources, rather than from meat. Here's why: Iron in plants is called *nonheme iron,* which is more absorbable when your body needs more and less absorbable when your body has plenty of iron already. That is important because if your body gets too much iron, it can be harmful to your heart and other organs.

Iron from meat is less desirable. When iron has been processed through a cow's body, it is called *heme iron.* Because your body cannot regulate the absorption of heme iron, over the long run you—and many meat-eaters—will accumulate too much iron.

So think "greens and beans," and you'll get not only calcium, but iron, too, in a form your body is designed to absorb and regulate.

FAT • You need just traces of fat in your diet, and that quantity is easily obtained from healthful plant sources. There is plenty of healthful fat in walnuts, soy products, flax seeds, and other foods. But let me make one more pitch for green vegetables: Although they do not contain much fat, the traces they do contain supply the healthy fats your body actually needs.

Animal products are often high in "bad" fat—that is, the *saturated fat* that raises cholesterol levels and is linked to Alzheimer's disease. It also packs into your cells and contributes to insulin resistance.

Although most plants contain modest quantities of fats—which is good—there are a few exceptions. Nuts, seeds, avocados, olives, and full-fat soy products are high in fat. While their fat is much healthier than the fat found in dairy products and meats (vegetable fats are generally much lower in saturated fat), these fats are still as high in calories as any other fat, so I would encourage you to keep consumption of these fatty foods to a minimum.

So there you have it. Eat a variety of vegetables, fruits, whole grains, and legumes. Avoid adding fats to your foods. Take a vitamin B_{12} supplement, and add a vitamin D supplement if you are not getting regular sunshine. Do that, and you've got complete nutrition.

BREAKFASTS

CHAMPION MUESLI

MAKES 4 SERVINGS

This is such a satisfying and wholesome breakfast, with just a touch of sweetness. The ultimate breakfast for champions!

2 cups rolled oats
¼ cup almond meal (or 3 tablespoons hemp seeds or 3 tablespoons tigernut meal for nut-free)
2 tablespoons sunflower seeds or pumpkin seeds (optional)

⅓ cup raisins
½ teaspoon cinnamon
¼ teaspoon nutmeg
Pinch of sea salt
1 large apple, grated (see Note)
2–2½ cups low-fat nondairy milk

In a large bowl, combine the oats, almond meal, seeds (if using), raisins, cinnamon, nutmeg, salt, apple, and 2 cups of the milk. Stir thoroughly. Cover and let the mixture soak overnight or for several hours. Serve, adding the remaining milk to achieve your desired consistency and topping with extra fruit, if you like.

NOTE • If you're soaking the muesli overnight, you can hold off on grating and adding the apple until the morning, if you like, to keep it fresher. If you'd like to add it ahead of time, toss the grated apple with a little lemon juice before mixing it in. Also try using apples that don't brown as easily, such as Ambrosia, Cameo, and Gala varieties.

NUTRITIONAL FACTS
Per serving: 304 calories, 9 g protein, 54 g carbohydrates, 17 g sugar, 7 g total fat, 20% calories from fat, 7 g fiber, 131 mg sodium

CREAMY PRESSURE-COOKED STEEL-CUT OATS

MAKES 5 SERVINGS

Steel-cut oats cook up fast in a pressure cooker or instant pot (and even faster when you use boiled water), and nondairy milk makes them extra creamy.

1½ cups steel-cut oats

3 cups boiled water

2 cups + ⅓–½ cup vanilla or plain low-fat nondairy milk

1 teaspoon cinnamon

½ teaspoon turmeric (optional)

¼ teaspoon ground nutmeg

A couple pinches of sea salt

⅔ cup raisins

Drizzle of coconut nectar or pure maple syrup (optional)

In a pressure cooker or instant pot, combine the oats, water, 2 cups of the milk, cinnamon, turmeric, nutmeg, and salt. Set it manually to cook for 7 to 9 minutes (see Note). When the oats are done cooking, turn off the pressure cooker and let the pressure release naturally. Remove the cover, stir in the raisins, and replace the cover. Let the oats sit for a couple of minutes to allow the raisins to plump up. Stir in the additional ⅓ to ½ cup milk to achieve the desired consistency, taste, and add extra cinnamon or nectar or syrup (if using). Serve.

NOTE • Steel cut oats can cook much faster than in 7 to 9 minutes in a pressure cooker, however they become much creamier with this cooking time. Cook them for 10 minutes for the creamiest texture.

NUTRITIONAL FACTS
Per serving: 296 calories, 9 g protein, 58 g carbohydrates, 17 g sugar, 4 g total fat, 12% calories from fat, 6 g fiber, 181 mg sodium

BLENDED BERRY OATS

MAKES 2 SERVINGS

Pop everything into the blender. Voilà, breakfast is served!

½ cup rolled oats

1 tablespoon ground chia seeds

4 or 5 pitted dates

⅛ teaspoon cinnamon or nutmeg

¼ teaspoon almond extract (optional)

Pinch of sea salt

1 cup + 2–3 tablespoons low-fat nondairy milk

1¼ cups raspberries, fresh or frozen (see Note)

In a blender, combine the oats, chia, dates, cinnamon, almond extract (if using), salt, and 1 cup of the milk. Puree until just combined. Add 1 cup of the raspberries and puree again just to combine. Transfer the mixture to a bowl or jar using a spatula, and stir in the remaining ¼ cup berries. Cover and refrigerate overnight (or for several hours, if eating as a snack). Before eating, add the additional 2 to 3 tablespoons of milk to thin, if desired.

NOTE • A mix of berries can be used here, such as a blend of blueberries, strawberries, and blackberries—whatever you like and have on hand.

NUTRITIONAL FACTS

Per serving: 267 calories, 8 g protein, 53 g carbohydrates, 20 g sugar, 5 g total fat, 15% calories from fat, 16 g fiber, 199 mg sodium

LOW-FAT GRANOLA

MAKES 6 SERVINGS

Farewell to store-bought granola! This one is far healthier and much lower in fat, but it packs plenty of flavor.

4 cups rolled oats	½ cup brown rice syrup
2 teaspoons cinnamon	⅓ cup unsweetened applesauce
¼ teaspoon sea salt	1 teaspoon pure vanilla extract
1 tablespoon cashew or almond butter	¼ cup raisins, dried cranberries, or other dried fruit
½ tablespoon blackstrap molasses	

Preheat the oven to 300°F. Line a large rimmed baking pan with a sheet of parchment paper.

In a large bowl, combine the oats, cinnamon, and salt, and stir to combine. In a blender, combine the nut butter, molasses, syrup, applesauce, and vanilla. Puree until smooth. Add the blended mixture to the oat mixture and stir to fully combine. Transfer the mixture to the prepared baking sheet. Bake for 25 minutes, stirring once. Turn off the heat, add the dried fruit, and let the granola sit in the warm oven for 10 to 15 minutes. Remove the baking pan, let the granola cool completely, and then break it into clusters and transfer it to an airtight container. Serve in a bowl with nondairy milk and fruit, or nibble on it as a snack.

Shown in color insert pages

NUTRITIONAL FACTS
Per serving: 346 calories, 8 g protein, 68 g carbohydrates, 22 g sugar, 5 g total fat, 12% calories from fat, 6 g fiber, 116 mg sodium

CINNAMON WISP PANCAKES

MAKES 4 SERVINGS

These golden, fluffy pancakes have a delightful hint of cinnamon.

2 cups oat flour	Pinch of sea salt
2 tablespoons chia seeds	1½ teaspoons vanilla extract
1 tablespoon baking powder	1¾ cups + ¼ cup vanilla low-fat nondairy milk
2 teaspoons cinnamon	

In a large bowl, combine the oat flour, chia seeds, baking powder, cinnamon, and salt. Stir to combine. Add the vanilla and 1¾ cups of the milk, and whisk through the dry mixture until combined. Let the batter sit for a few minutes to thicken.

Lightly coat a large nonstick skillet with cooking spray. Heat the pan over medium-high heat for a few minutes until hot, then reduce the heat to medium or medium-low and let it rest for a minute. Using a ladle, scoop ¼ to ⅓ cup of the batter into the pan for each pancake. Depending on the size of pan, cook 2 or 3 pancakes at a time. Cook for several minutes, until small bubbles form on the outer edges and in the centers and the pancakes start to look dry on the top. (Wait until those bubbles form, or the pancakes will be tricky to flip.) Once ready, flip the pancakes to lightly cook the other side for about a minute. Repeat until the batter is all used, adding the extra milk, 1 tablespoon at a time, if needed to thin the batter as you go.

Shown in color insert pages

NUTRITIONAL FACTS
Per serving: 312 calories, 11 g protein, 54 g carbohydrates, 5 g sugar, 6 g total fat, 17% calories from fat, 9 g fiber, 483 mg sodium

RICE BREAKFAST BAKE

MAKES 4 SERVINGS

Cook extra rice for dinner so you can make this breakfast later in the week. It makes a great dessert, too.

1¼ cups vanilla low-fat nondairy milk

1 tablespoon ground chia seeds

2½ cups cooked short-grain brown rice

2 cups sliced ripe (but not overripe) banana (2–2½ medium bananas)

1 cup chopped apple

2–3 tablespoons raisins (optional)

1 teaspoon cinnamon

½ teaspoon pure vanilla extract

¼ teaspoon freshly grated nutmeg (optional)

Rounded ⅛ teaspoon sea salt

2 tablespoons almond meal (or 1 tablespoon tigernut flour, for nut-free option)

2 tablespoons coconut sugar

Preheat the oven to 400°F.

In a blender or food processor, combine the milk, ground chia, and 1 cup of the rice. Puree until fairly smooth. In a large bowl, combine the blended mixture, bananas, apple, raisins (if using), cinnamon, vanilla, nutmeg (if using), salt, and the remaining 1½ cups rice. Stir to fully combine. Transfer the mixture to a baking dish (8" x 8" or similar size). In a small bowl, combine the almond meal and sugar, and sprinkle it over the rice mixture. Cover with foil and bake for 15 minutes, then remove the foil and bake for another 5 minutes. Remove, let cool for 5 to 10 minutes, then serve.

NUTRITIONAL FACTS

Per serving: 334 calories, 7 g protein, 69 g carbohydrates, 22 g sugar, 5 g total fat, 12% calories from fat, 7 g fiber, 145 mg sodium

ORANGE-BERRY PANCAKE SYRUP

MAKES 8 SERVINGS (2 CUPS)

Blending berries into maple syrup makes a flavorful pancake topping and a great dessert sauce, as well.

2 cups raspberries, fresh or frozen

½ cup fresh orange juice (see Note)

¼ cup pure maple syrup

Pinch of sea salt

In a blender, combine the raspberries, juice, syrup, and salt. Puree until smooth, stopping to scrape down the blender as needed. If the mixture is too thick (particularly if using frozen berries), you may need to scrape down more often or add a tablespoon or two of water to assist with the blending. Once it's smooth, transfer the syrup to a jar or other airtight container and store it in the refrigerator. It keeps for about a week in the fridge.

NOTE • The orange juice helps sweeten this sauce without using too much maple syrup. If you're unsure of how you'll like the flavor, start with about ¼ cup of orange juice, and adjust to taste, also adding more maple syrup as desired.

Shown in color insert pages

NUTRITIONAL FACTS
Per serving: 65 calories, 1 g protein, 16 g carbohydrates, 10 g sugar, 0.4 g total fat, 6% calories from fat, 4 g fiber, 38 mg sodium

SWEET POTATO BREAKFAST BITES

MAKES 12

Sweet potatoes bring natural sweetness to these miniature muffin-like snacks.

1½ cups precooked and cooled sweet potato (see Note)

½ cup pure maple syrup

1 teaspoon pure vanilla extract

1¼ cups rolled oats

1 cup oat flour

½ teaspoon cinnamon

½ teaspoon pumpkin pie spice (optional; can substitute another ½ teaspoon cinnamon)

2 teaspoons baking powder

¼ teaspoon sea salt

2–3 tablespoons raisins or sugar-free nondairy chocolate chips (optional)

Preheat the oven to 350°F and line a baking sheet with parchment paper.

In a medium bowl, mash the sweet potato. Add the syrup and vanilla and stir to combine. Add the oats, oat flour, cinnamon, pumpkin pie spice (if using), baking powder, and salt, and mix until well combined. Add the raisins or chips (if using), and stir to combine. Refrigerate for 5 to 10 minutes. Scoop 1½-tablespoon rounds of the mixture onto the parchment, spacing them 1 to 2 inches apart. Bake for 17 to 18 minutes, or until set to the touch. Remove from the oven, and let cool.

NOTE • It's always helpful to have precooked sweet potato in the fridge. It will keep for 5 to 6 days to use in recipes. Baking brings out the best flavor and is very easy to do. Just place whole sweet potatoes on a baking sheet lined with parchment paper. Bake at 450°F for 40 to 60 minutes, or until very soft. (Cooking time will depend on the size of the sweet potato.) To measure, you just need to remove the peel and break up the sweet potato into a measuring cup.

NUTRITIONAL FACTS
Per 2–Breakfast Bite serving: 251 calories, 6 g protein, 52 g carbohydrates, 19 g sugar, 2 g total fat, 8% calories from fat, 5 g fiber, 281 mg sodium

AMARANTH PORRIDGE

MAKES 2 SERVINGS

Amaranth marries oat flour or almond meal to create a hearty, satisfying, and tasty porridge.

⅓ cup amaranth

1 cup water

1 cup vanilla low-fat nondairy milk

¼–½ teaspoon cinnamon

Couple pinches of freshly grated nutmeg (or cardamom, for a spicier flavor)

Pinch of sea salt

⅓ cup oat flour (see Note to substitute almond meal)

1–2 tablespoons maple syrup

Fresh berries or other fruit (optional; see Optional Toppings)

In a small pot over high heat, combine the amaranth, water, milk, cinnamon, nutmeg, and salt. Bring to a boil, then reduce the heat to low and let simmer, covered, for 25 minutes, stirring once or twice. Whisk in the oat flour and cook over low heat for a minute or two. Stir until thick and smooth. Turn off the heat, adjust the seasoning to taste with extra cinnamon or nutmeg, and add the syrup to taste. Serve, topped with berries or fruit (if using).

NOTE • If you cannot use oat products, try almond meal. Follow the recipe, but substitute ½ cup + 1 to 2 tablespoons almond meal (enough to thicken) for the oat flour. Stir, uncovered, over low heat for a few minutes, until the porridge is bubbling and thick. It will take a little longer to thicken with the almond meal than with the oat flour. You can also add 1 tablespoon of ground chia seeds to thicken the porridge and add even more nutrients. Season with extra cinnamon, nutmeg, and pure maple syrup, coconut nectar, or coconut sugar to taste.

OPTIONAL TOPPINGS

- Add in dried fruit, like chopped dates, raisins, cranberries, bananas, or apricots!
- Add frozen berries straight to the hot oatmeal to help cool it instantly.
- In summer, add in fresh berries or chopped peaches or nectarines.
- In fall and winter, add in chopped apples or pears.

NUTRITIONAL FACTS
Per serving: 281 calories, 9 g protein, 52 g carbohydrates, 12 g sugar, 5 g total fat, 14% calories from fat, 5 g fiber, 198 mg sodium

BREAKFAST POLENTA CAKES

MAKES 2 SERVINGS

With the convenience of prepared polenta, you'll have a fun and simple twist on pancakes: polenta cakes!

1 tube (18 ounces or similar size) prepared, plain, organic polenta

1 teaspoon cinnamon

½ cup Orange-Berry Pancake Syrup (page 30) or Orange-Mango Cream (page 194)

Optional: sliced bananas, fresh berries, sliced peaches or apples

Place a nonstick skillet over medium-high heat. Slice a tube of polenta into discs about ½" thick. (This should yield 17 or 18 slices.) Place the cinnamon on a plate, and dredge the polenta slices through the cinnamon to coat, dusting off excess as you go. Place the polenta slices in the heated pan, working in batches (unless you have a very large skillet to accommodate all slices). Cook for about 5 minutes on the first side, then turn and cook for another 4 to 5 minutes on the second side, until both sides are a little golden. Serve, layering with fruit (if using) and topping with the Orange-Berry Pancake Syrup or Orange-Mango Cream.

NUTRITIONAL FACTS

Per serving (with Orange-Berry Syrup): 227 calories, 4 g protein, 51 g carbohydrates, 11 g sugar, 1 g total fat, 4% calories from fat, 6 g fiber, 374 mg sodium

Per serving (with Orange-Mango Cream): 219 calories, 4 g protein, 43 g carbohydrates, 7 g sugar, 3 g total fat, 12% calories from fat, 3 g fiber, 386 mg sodium

SWEET POTATO TOASTS

MAKES 1 SERVING

Elevate everyday toast with the addition of deliciously satisfying sweet potato. Feel free to add plenty of pepper and additional lemon juice for an additional savory boost!

2 slices sprouted grain bread	A couple pinches of sea salt
½ cup mashed cooked sweet potato, peel removed (see Note)	Freshly ground black pepper (optional)
½–1 teaspoon lemon juice	2 tablespoons cubed avocado or 1 tablespoon sliced black olives

Toast the bread. In a small bowl, mash the sweet potato with the lemon juice (adjusting to taste), salt, and pepper (if using). Distribute the mashed sweet potato between the slices of toast, and top with either the cubed avocado or the black olives. Serve!

NOTE • It's useful to bake sweet potatoes in advance. Place whole sweet potatoes on a baking sheet lined with parchment. Bake at 450°F for 40 to 60 minutes, or until very soft. (Cooking time will depend on the size of the sweet potato.) Store in the fridge until ready to use (up to 6 days) or in the freezer for a couple of months.

Shown in color insert pages

NUTRITIONAL FACTS
Per serving: 312 calories, 8 g protein, 59 g carbohydrates, 11 g sugar, 5 g total fat, 14% calories from fat, 8 g fiber, 1,018 mg sodium

OVERNIGHT BERRY OATS

MAKES 2 SERVINGS

Frozen berries add a boost of flavor and color to overnight oats. This dish is perfect for a quick breakfast or a satisfying afternoon or evening snack.

1   cup rolled oats

1   cup raspberries or mixed berries (such as blueberries, strawberries, and blackberries), fresh or frozen

1   cup + 1–2 tablespoons low-fat nondairy milk (plus more for serving, if desired)

½   tablespoon chia seeds

2   tablespoons coconut nectar or pure maple syrup

    Pinch of sea salt

In a bowl or large jar, combine the oats, berries, milk, chia seeds, nectar or syrup, and salt. Cover and refrigerate overnight (or for at least several hours). Serve with more milk to thin, if desired, and also try some additional add-ins (see Note).

NOTE • When serving, you can add other toppings, including more berries, sliced ripe banana, a sprinkle of cocoa nibs, or 1 to 2 tablespoons of hemp or pumpkin seeds.

NUTRITIONAL FACTS
Per serving: 326 calories, 9 g protein, 64 g carbohydrates, 21 g sugar, 5 g total fat, 13% calories from fat, 14 g fiber, 205 mg sodium

BAKED OATMEAL CUPS

MAKES 15

Take your oatmeal on the go! Grab a couple of these oatmeal cups to tackle your morning appetite in a nutritious way.

3 cups rolled oats

½ cup oat flour

3 tablespoons flax meal

1 teaspoon cinnamon

Rounded ⅛ teaspoon sea salt

2 cups sliced overripe banana

⅓ cup brown rice syrup (see Note)

⅓ cup raisins

2 tablespoons sugar-free nondairy chocolate chips (optional)

Line a muffin pan with 15 parchment cupcake liners. Preheat the oven to 350°F.

In a large mixing bowl, combine the oats, oat flour, flax meal, cinnamon, and salt. Stir to combine. Mash or puree the banana using a food processor or immersion blender. Add the banana, syrup, raisins, and chips (if using). Stir until thoroughly combined. Using a cookie scoop, place ¼ to ⅓ cup of the batter in each muffin cup. Use a spatula or your fingers to lightly pack in the mixture. (Dampen your fingers to make it easier.) Bake for 20 minutes. Remove and let cool in the pan for about 5 minutes, then transfer to a cooling rack. Enjoy warm or cooled. Store in an airtight container in the fridge.

NOTE • Don't substitute maple syrup here; it's not thick and sticky enough. Coconut palm nectar and barley malt syrup are acceptable alternatives to brown rice syrup.

NUTRITIONAL FACTS

Per Oatmeal Cup: 133 calories, 3 g protein, 27 g carbohydrates, 7 g sugar, 2 g total fat, 13% calories from fat, 3 g fiber, 37 mg sodium

POLENTA PORRIDGE WITH BERRY SWIRL

MAKES 4 SERVINGS

This creamy porridge has a vibrant pop of color and flavor, thanks to the raspberry swirl.

1 cup frozen raspberries

¼ cup + 1 tablespoon pure maple syrup

2 cups vanilla or plain low-fat nondairy milk

1 cup water

¼ teaspoon nutmeg

Couple pinches of sea salt

1 cup cornmeal

1 cup fresh berries for serving or 1 cup sliced ripe banana (optional)

Sprinkle of coconut sugar for serving (optional)

In a blender, combine the raspberries and ¼ cup of the syrup. Blend until pureed. In a saucepan over medium-high heat, bring the milk, water, nutmeg, and salt to a boil. Reduce the heat to medium and slowly whisk in the cornmeal. Stir frequently for about 5 minutes, until the cornmeal comes to a slow bubble and thickens. Add the remaining 1 tablespoon syrup and stir to combine. Remove from the heat. Pour the porridge into bowls, and add the raspberry sauce, swirling it through the porridge with a butter knife or spoon. Serve, topping with the berries or banana (if using) and a sprinkle of coconut sugar (if using).

NOTE • If polenta sits for some time on the stove after cooking, it will continue to thicken. To thin it again, stir in extra milk over low heat.

NUTRITIONAL FACTS
Per serving: 300 calories, 6 g protein, 65 g carbohydrates, 23 g sugar, 2 g total fat, 6% calories from fat, 6 g fiber, 207 mg sodium

CINNAMON BUN OATMEAL

MAKES 3 SERVINGS

The combination of cinnamon, dates, and raisins turns this oatmeal into a cinnamon bun in a bowl!

1½ cups rolled oats (see Note)	3 tablespoons raisins
⅓ cup chopped dates	¾ cup + 1–2 tablespoons low-fat nondairy milk
1 teaspoon cinnamon	
Pinch of sea salt (optional)	Sprinkle of cinnamon
2 cups water	3 teaspoons coconut sugar (optional)

In a pot over high heat, combine the oats, dates, cinnamon, salt, and water, and bring to a boil. Reduce the heat to low and let simmer for 7 to 8 minutes, until the water is absorbed and the oats are softening. Add the raisins and ¾ cup of the milk, and cook for another 6 to 7 minutes, or until the raisins have softened. Remove from the heat and let stand for a few minutes. The oatmeal will thicken more as it sits, so add the remaining 1 to 2 tablespoons of milk if needed to thin. Top each serving with the cinnamon and 1 teaspoon of the coconut sugar (if using).

NOTE • Rolled oats can vary in thickness. Some are smaller and thinner (more like quick oats) and others are heftier, as we'd expect with rolled oats. Because of that, cooking time can vary slightly, with thicker oats requiring a longer cooking time and a little extra milk.

NUTRITIONAL FACTS
Per serving: 251 calories, 7 g protein, 51 g carbohydrates, 18 g sugar, 3 g total fat, 11% calories from fat, 7 g fiber, 34 mg sodium

BERRY "SCUFFINS"

MAKES 9

What do you get when you cross a scone with a muffin? A scuffin, of course! These are easy to make and just delightful during berry season.

1½ cups oat flour

¾ cup rolled oats

1 teaspoon baking powder

½ teaspoon baking soda

¼ teaspoon sea salt

1 teaspoon lemon zest

½ cup plain nondairy yogurt (see Yogurt Note)

½ cup pure maple syrup

3–5 tablespoons low-fat nondairy milk (see Milk Note)

½ cup blueberries, strawberries (cut into pieces), or raspberries (see Berry Note)

Preheat the oven to 350°F. Line a large baking sheet with parchment paper.

In a large bowl, combine the flour, oats, baking powder, baking soda, salt, and lemon zest. In a small bowl, whisk together the yogurt, syrup, and milk until well combined. Add the wet mixture to the dry, folding in until just nicely combined. Add the berries, and gently fold them in so they don't bleed too much color. Using an ice cream scoop, place mounds of the batter (3 to 4 tablespoons each) on your baking sheet, spacing them 1 to 2 inches apart, to make 9 "scuffins." Bake for 15 to 16 minutes, or until set. (Gently touch one in the center; it should be firm to the touch.) Remove from the oven, let cool for a minute or two on the pan, and then transfer to a cooling rack to cool completely.

YOGURT NOTE • If you only have vanilla yogurt, you can use it, but reduce the maple syrup so the scuffins aren't too sweet. Use ⅓ cup maple syrup, and make up the extra couple of table-spoons with milk.

MILK NOTE • How much milk you use will depend on the consistency of your brand of nondairy yogurt. Some brands are quite dense and thick, so you may find you need as much as 5 tablespoons of milk. Other dairy-free yogurts are much thinner, and you may need just 3 tablespoons of milk. Start with 3 when whisking the wet ingredients together, and then, if the mixture is very stiff, add the additional 1 to 2 tablespoons of milk when folding in.

BERRY NOTE • If you're using frozen berries, your baking time may be a little longer. Test, and bake for another minute or two if needed to set. If you use raspberries, the color will bleed a little more, but the flavor is delicious!

NUTRITIONAL FACTS
Per Scuffin: 163 calories, 4 g protein, 33 g carbohydrates, 13 g sugar, 2 g total fat, 11% calories from fat, 3 g fiber, 197 mg sodium

MI-SO LOVE AVOCADO TOAST!

MAKES 1 SERVING

A light spread of miso makes this easy meal irresistible.

2 slices sprouted grain bread (see Note)

1–1½ teaspoons chickpea miso (or other mild-flavored miso)

¼ cup ripe avocado, mashed

Squeeze of lemon juice (about ½ teaspoon)

A couple pinches of sea salt

1 teaspoon nutritional yeast (optional)

Freshly ground black pepper to taste

2 thick slices ripe tomato, or a handful of chopped lettuce or baby spinach

Toast the bread. While it's still warm, spread about ½ teaspoon of the miso on each slice. Distribute the avocado over the miso, and add a squeeze of lemon juice and a pinch of salt. Sprinkle on nutritional yeast (if using), and pepper. Top with the sliced tomatoes, lettuce, or spinach.

NOTE • For breakfast, one slice may be sufficient, depending upon your appetite. Serve with fresh fruit, such as a navel orange, fresh berries, or sliced melon. For lunch, instead of tomato or greens, sprinkle ⅓ cup of Teriyaki Chickpeas (page 185) or Moroccan-Roasted Chickpeas (page 188) on top of the toast and serve with a green salad or crudité, such as spears of cucumbers and carrots.

Shown in color insert pages

NUTRITIONAL FACTS
Per serving: 250 calories, 7 g protein, 38 g carbohydrates, 4 g sugar, 8 g total fat, 28% calories from fat, 6 g fiber, 1,190 mg sodium

LEMON-PINEAPPLE MUFFINS

MAKES 12

Fluffy, light, and fragrant—these muffins will become a favorite!

2 cups oat flour

1 cup spelt flour

⅓ cup coconut sugar

2½ teaspoons baking powder

½ teaspoon baking soda

½ teaspoon cinnamon

¼ teaspoon nutmeg

Generous ¼ teaspoon sea salt

1–1½ teaspoons lemon zest

¾ cup plain nondairy yogurt

¼ cup coconut nectar or maple syrup

1½ tablespoons freshly squeezed lemon juice

1 cup plain low-fat nondairy milk

1 cup diced fresh, frozen, or canned pineapple

Preheat the oven to 350°F. Line a muffin pan with 12 parchment cupcake liners (see Note).

In a large bowl, combine the oat flour, spelt flour, and sugar. Sift in the baking powder and baking soda, then add the cinnamon, nutmeg, salt, and lemon zest. Stir to combine. In a small bowl, combine the yogurt with the nectar or syrup, lemon juice, and milk. Add the wet mixture to the dry, stirring until just combined, and then gently fold in the pineapple. Pour the mixture into the muffin cups. Bake for 26 to 28 minutes, or until a toothpick inserted in the center of a muffin comes out clean. Remove from the oven, cool for a couple of minutes in the pan, and then transfer the muffins to a cooling rack.

NOTE • These are larger, "bakery-style" muffins, so expect to fully fill those muffin liners!

Shown in color insert pages

NUTRITIONAL FACTS
Per muffin: 175 calories, 5 g protein, 36 g carbohydrates, 13 g sugar, 2 g total fat, 10% calories from fat, 4 g fiber, 240 mg sodium

COCOA CARROT MUFFINS

MAKES 12

These muffins have just the right amount of sweetness for a lovely breakfast.

2 cups spelt flour (or 1¾ cups whole wheat pastry flour)

⅓ cup coconut sugar (see Note)

¼ cup cocoa powder

1 teaspoon cinnamon

½ teaspoon nutmeg

¼ teaspoon sea salt

2 teaspoons baking powder

½ teaspoon baking soda

2 tablespoons nut butter, such as almond or cashew butter (or 1½ tablespoons tahini mixed with 1 tablespoon maple syrup)

1 cup low-fat nondairy milk

¾ cup unsweetened applesauce

1 cup grated carrot

¼ cup raisins

2 tablespoons sugar-free nondairy chocolate chips (optional)

Preheat the oven to 350°F. Line a muffin pan with 12 parchment cupcake liners.

In a large bowl, combine the flour, sugar, cocoa, cinnamon, nutmeg, salt, baking powder, and baking soda, stirring well. In a medium bowl, combine the nut butter with a few tablespoons of the milk, whisking it to incorporate fully. Continue to add the remaining milk and then the applesauce, stirring thoroughly. Add this wet mixture to the dry, along with the carrot, raisins, and chips (if using). Fold and mix until just combined; do not overmix. Spoon the batter into the cupcake liners. Bake for 23 to 24 minutes, or until a toothpick inserted in the center comes out clean. Remove from the oven, let cool in the pan for a couple of minutes, then transfer to a cooling rack.

NOTE • As explained above, these muffins are not overly sweet. If you think you'd like a touch more sweetness, try the batter after mixing and add another 2 to 4 teaspoons of sugar or another sprinkle of raisins!

Shown in color insert pages

NUTRITIONAL FACTS
Per muffin: 137 calories, 4 g protein, 28 g carbohydrates, 11 g sugar, 2 g total fat, 15% calories from fat, 4 g fiber, 205 mg sodium

BLUEBERRY CORNMEAL MUFFINS

MAKES 12

These tender, fragrant muffins are perfect for breakfast, snacks, or tea with friends.

2 cups oat flour

½ cup fine corn flour (see Note)

¼ cup coconut sugar

2 teaspoons baking powder

½ teaspoon baking soda

¼ teaspoon sea salt

1 teaspoon lemon zest

½ cup + 2–3 tablespoons plain nondairy yogurt

¼ cup pure maple syrup

½ cup plain low-fat nondairy milk

1 teaspoon lemon juice or apple cider vinegar

1 cup frozen or fresh blueberries

1 tablespoon oat flour

Preheat the oven to 350°F. Line a muffin pan with 12 parchment cupcake liners.

In a large bowl, combine the oat flour, corn flour, sugar, baking powder, baking soda, salt, and lemon zest. Stir well. In a medium bowl, combine the yogurt, syrup, milk, and lemon juice or apple cider vinegar, and stir to combine. Add the wet ingredients to the dry and mix until just combined. Toss the berries with the oat flour, and fold them into the batter. Spoon the batter into the muffin liners. Bake for 25 minutes. Remove from the oven and let the muffins cool in the pan for a couple of minutes, then transfer to a cooling rack.

NOTE • Corn flour is a finer grind than cornmeal, which is used for polenta.

Shown in color insert pages

NUTRITIONAL FACTS
Per muffin: 152 calories, 4 g protein, 31 g carbohydrates, 11 g sugar, 2 g total fat, 11% calories from fat, 3 g fiber, 191 mg sodium

ENCHANTED SMOOTHIE BOWL

MAKES 3 SERVINGS

Start your morning with this enchanting deep purple, nutrient-rich smoothie bowl!

1½ cups frozen blueberries

1 cup frozen raspberries

1 cup sliced frozen or room-temperature overripe banana

2 cups baby spinach leaves

1 tablespoon orange juice

2–3 tablespoons vanilla protein powder (optional)

1 cup + 2–3 tablespoons water or nondairy milk (for a creamy texture)

½ cup sliced ripe banana

½ cup seasonal fruit, such as sliced kiwi, sliced strawberries, chopped pear, or clementine segments

In a blender, combine the blueberries, raspberries, banana, spinach, juice, protein powder (if using), and 1 cup of the water or milk, and puree. Add the remaining water or milk 1 tablespoon at a time if needed to thin, but only add as much as is needed to be able to blend, so the mixture stays very thick. Divide among 3 bowls and top with the banana and seasonal fruit.

Shown in color insert pages

NUTRITIONAL FACTS

Per serving: 275 calories, 5 g protein, 67 g carbohydrates, 37 g sugar, 2 g total fat, 7% calories from fat, 15 g fiber, 25 mg sodium

GREEN NICE CREAM BREAKFAST BOWL

MAKES 3 SERVINGS

Ever want ice cream for breakfast? With whole fruit and spinach, you can have this ice cream any time of day.

- 3 cups sliced, frozen, overripe banana
- 1 cup frozen pineapple chunks
- 2 cups baby spinach
  Flesh of 1 ripe avocado (about ½ cup)
  Pinch of sea salt

- 3–5 tablespoons low-fat nondairy milk
- 1–2 tablespoons coconut syrup (optional)
  - ½ cup fresh sliced banana
  - ½ cup fresh berries

In a blender or food processor, combine the banana, pineapple, spinach, avocado, salt, and 3 tablespoons of the milk. Puree until very smooth. If the mixture is stubborn and not blending, add the additional 2 tablespoons of milk as needed to get the mixture moving. Taste, and add the syrup if desired to sweeten. Spoon the mixture into 3 serving bowls, and top with the banana and berries.

NUTRITIONAL FACTS
Per serving: 337 calories, 5 g protein, 70 g carbohydrates, 37 g sugar, 8 g total fat, 20% calories from fat, 12 g fiber, 126 mg sodium

CAULIFLOWER SCRAMBLE

MAKES 3 SERVINGS

This savory breakfast can double as lunch or dinner. It's very satisfying and easy to make.

1 package (12–16 ounces) medium or medium-firm tofu

3½–4 cups steamed cauliflower florets, lightly mashed (see Cauliflower Note)

½ teaspoon onion powder

½ teaspoon garlic powder

½ teaspoon sea salt

¼ teaspoon prepared mustard

½ teaspoon black salt (or another ¼ teaspoon sea salt; see Black Salt Note)

½ tablespoon tahini

2½–3 tablespoons nutritional yeast

2–3 cups chopped spinach or kale

In a large nonstick skillet, use your fingers to crumble the tofu, breaking it up well. Place the skillet over medium heat. Add the cauliflower, onion powder, garlic powder, sea salt, mustard, and black salt. Cook for 3 to 4 minutes, then add the tahini and nutritional yeast and stir to combine thoroughly. If the mixture is sticking, add 1 to 2 tablespoons water. Add the spinach or kale during the final minutes of cooking, stirring until just nicely wilted and still bright green. Taste, season as desired, and serve.

CAULIFLOWER NOTE • Steaming the cauliflower helps it break down nicely for this scramble. You can steam it a day or two ahead of time to help speed preparation.

BLACK SALT NOTE • Black salt is not actually black in color, but rather is a light pink. It is sometimes labeled "kala namak" and it contributes an "eggy" flavor to the scramble. If you don't have it, simply omit and season with additional sea salt to taste, using a total of about ½ to ¾ teaspoon of salt. Black salt has a flavor that's both savory and salty, so use less sea salt if substituting.

IDEAS: For other add-ins, try a handful of chopped green onions or chives, 1 to 2 tablespoons of sliced olives, or ¼ cup of chopped sun-dried tomatoes.

NUTRITIONAL FACTS
Per serving: 196 calories, 21 g protein, 16 g carbohydrates, 3 g sugar, 9 g total fat, 37% calories from fat, 10 g fiber, 862 mg sodium

QUICK-ADILLAS

MAKES 2 SERVINGS

These are not quesadillas in the traditional sense. Still, it shows how a quick and delicious lunch can be prepped using some common ingredients and whole grain tortillas.

½ cup cooked white beans

⅓–½ cup cubed avocado

1 tablespoon lemon juice

½ tablespoon miso

¼ teaspoon smoked paprika

⅛ teaspoon sea salt

2 whole grain tortillas

½ cup thinly sliced red bell pepper or ⅓ cup chopped fresh spinach (or both)

¼ cup chopped fresh basil (optional)

In a bowl, coarsely mash the white beans, avocado, lemon juice, miso, smoked paprika, and sea salt. Stir through to combine. Spread about half the mixture on one tortilla. Top with the bell pepper/spinach, and basil, if using. Spread remaining mixture on the other tortilla. Sandwich the tortillas together. Place a nonstick skillet over medium-high heat. Put the quesadilla in the skillet and cook for about 3 minutes, until lightly browned. Flip and cook for 2 to 3 minutes, until lightly browned. The tortillas should be crisp, with the filling warmed inside, but it doesn't have to be hot. Transfer to a rack (so the underside doesn't soften) to cool slightly, then transfer to a plate and cut into wedges. Serve warm.

Shown in color insert pages

NUTRITIONAL FACTS
Per serving: 258 calories, 10 g protein, 41 g carbohydrate, 2 g sugar, 8 g total fat, 25% calories from fat, 9 g fiber, 751 mg sodium

DRINKS

TURMERIC MILK

MAKES 1 SERVING

A warm drink to tame the winter chill, boosted with nutritional spices.

1 cup plain low-fat nondairy milk

¼–½ teaspoon ground turmeric (adjust to taste)

¼ teaspoon ground cinnamon

¼ teaspoon ground ginger

Couple pinches of ground cardamom (optional)

Pinch or two of stevia or ½–1 tablespoon coconut nectar

In a small saucepan over medium to medium-high heat, combine the milk, turmeric, cinnamon, ginger, cardamom (if using), and a pinch of stevia or ½ tablespoon of nectar. Whisk until the milk is heated through. (This should only take a few minutes, so keep an eye on the milk so it doesn't boil over or scorch.) Once warmed through, pour into a mug. Taste, and if you'd like it a little sweeter, add the remaining stevia or coconut nectar.

Shown in color insert pages

NUTRITIONAL FACTS
Per serving: 97 calories, 4 g protein, 17 g carbohydrates, 7 g sugar, 2 g total fat, 14% calories from fat, 2 g fiber, 91 mg sodium

VANILLA GREEN TEA LATTE

MAKES 1 LARGE SERVING

Skip that pricey coffee house matcha latte, and make this in just minutes at home.

1¼ cups plain or vanilla low-fat nondairy milk

2 teaspoons matcha green tea powder + extra for garnish (optional)

3–4 tablespoons water

¼ teaspoon stevia powder or ½ tablespoon coconut nectar

⅛ teaspoon vanilla bean powder (see Note)

1 teaspoon coconut sugar (optional)

In a small saucepan over medium or medium-high heat, warm the milk. Whisk, allowing the milk to heat through and start to simmer. Meanwhile, in a small bowl or wide-mouthed mug, use a small whisk to combine 2 teaspoons of the matcha powder with the water. (It's helpful to sift the matcha first, but it's not essential if you whisk well.) Transfer the blended mix to a mug. Once the milk is gently bubbling at a low simmer, add a scant ¼ teaspoon of the stevia or ½ tablespoon of the nectar and the vanilla bean powder. Quickly whisk through and remove from the heat. Pour the milk into your mug with the matcha mix. (If you have a frother, you can froth the milk before pouring it into the mug.) Taste, and if you'd like a little extra sweetener, add additional stevia or nectar to taste. Sprinkle with the coconut sugar (if using) and a dusting of matcha powder (if using).

NOTE • The vanilla bean powder is not essential. You could also use the seeds scraped from a vanilla bean. But don't use vanilla extract in this recipe. If you don't have the powder or bean, simply omit the vanilla entirely.

NUTRITIONAL FACTS
Per serving: 117 calories, 5 g protein, 19 g carbohydrates, 9 g sugar, 2 g total fat, 14% calories from fat, 1 g fiber, 116 mg sodium

STRAWBERRIES 'N' CREAM SMOOTHIE

MAKES 2 SERVINGS (ABOUT 4 CUPS)

Blend this up when you'd like something sweet, nutritious, and satisfying!

2½–3 cups frozen strawberries

2 cups plain low-fat nondairy milk (can add more to thin if desired)

1 cup sliced, overripe, frozen banana

¼ teaspoon vanilla bean powder (optional)

½–1 tablespoon coconut nectar or pure maple syrup (optional)

In a blender, combine the strawberries, milk, banana, and vanilla bean powder (if using). Puree until smooth. Taste, and add the nectar or syrup (if using) to sweeten to taste. Serve.

Shown in color insert pages

NUTRITIONAL FACTS

Per serving: 252 calories, 6 g protein, 57 g carbohydrates, 29 g sugar, 2 g total fat, 7% calories from fat, 9 g fiber, 97 mg sodium

BIG GREEN SMOOTHIE

MAKES 2 SERVINGS

This smoothie packs nutrient power for a healthy snack or breakfast on the go.

3 cups packed baby spinach (see Spinach Note)

½ cup sliced overripe banana, fresh or frozen

½ cup sliced or cubed cucumber (see Cucumber Note)

¼ cup fresh parsley leaves (optional)

1 lemon, peeled (can leave whole, seeds intact)

1–2 tablespoons hemp seeds (optional)

1–1½ cups frozen mango cubes

¾–1 cup water

In a blender, combine the spinach, banana, cucumber, parsley (if using), lemon, hemp seeds (if using), 1 cup of the mango, and ¾ cup of the water. Puree until very smooth. Add the extra ¼ cup of water if needed to thin, and add the additional ½ cup mango to sweeten to taste.

SPINACH NOTE • If you are new to green smoothies, start with a mild green like spinach or lettuce. Then you can try incorporating stronger-tasting greens, such as kale and collards, adjusting the quantity to taste as needed.

CUCUMBER NOTE • It's helpful to stock up on organic cucumbers when they are on special, then slice them thickly and store them in the freezer to use in smoothies.

Shown in color insert pages

NUTRITIONAL FACTS

Per serving: 106 calories, 3 g protein, 26 g carbohydrates, 17 g sugar, 1 g total fat, 6% calories from fat, 4 g fiber, 41 mg sodium

CREAMSICLE SMOOTHIE

MAKES 2 LARGE SERVINGS (ABOUT 3½ CUPS)

The creamy deliciousness of the classic Creamsicle frozen treat in a smoothie!

- 1 large orange, peeled (can substitute ½ cup orange juice)
- 1 small lemon (or ½ large lemon), peeled
- ½ cup sliced raw carrots
- 1 cup + 1–2 tablespoons low-fat nondairy milk
- ½ cup cubed frozen pineapple or frozen mango
- 1 cup sliced, frozen, overripe banana (see Note)
- 1–3 tablespoons vanilla protein powder (optional)
- ½ cup ice (optional)

In a blender, combine the orange, lemon, carrots, milk, pineapple or mango, banana, and 1 tablespoon of the protein powder (if using). Puree until very smooth. Taste, and add the remaining 2 tablespoons protein powder, if desired, as well as the additional 1 to 2 tablespoons milk to thin, if desired. Divide the ice (if using) between 2 glasses, and pour the smoothie over the ice. Serve.

NOTE • The quantities of pineapple, banana, and mango can be changed if you prefer one more than the others and want to change the flavor of the smoothie slightly. For instance, you can use 1 cup of frozen mango and ½ cup of pineapple, or ¾ cup of frozen banana and ¾ cup of frozen pineapple. Be sure to use frozen for a thick smoothie.

NUTRITIONAL FACTS
Per serving: 193 calories, 4 g protein, 45 g carbohydrates, 27 g sugar, 1 g total fat, 6% calories from fat, 7 g fiber, 68 mg sodium

SUGAR-FREE LEMONADE

MAKES 3 SERVINGS

Lemonade is so refreshing. This homemade version is sugar-free and simple to make!

4	cups water	¾–1	cup ice cubes
⅓	cup fresh lemon juice (see Note)	½	cup fresh or frozen raspberries
¾–1	teaspoon stevia powder		

In a jug or pitcher, combine the water, lemon juice, and ¾ teaspoon of the stevia, whisking to incorporate. Adjust to taste with the remaining ¼ teaspoon stevia, if desired. Chill. Divide the ice and raspberries among 3 glasses, pour in the lemonade, and serve.

NOTE • You could substitute an equal amount of lime juice for the lemon juice to make Sugar-Free Limeade.

NUTRITIONAL FACTS
Per serving: 18 calories, 0 g protein, 5 g carbohydrates, 2 g sugar, 0.2 g total fat, 9% calories from fat, 2 g fiber, 13 mg sodium

FRUIT SPRITZER

MAKES 1 SERVING

A light homemade soda-spritzer—perfect for summer and holiday parties, too!

1 cup sparkling mineral water

½ cup pure cranberry, pomegranate, or cherry juice (see Juice Note)

Few pinches of stevia (see Stevia Note)

½ cup ice cubes

Lemon, lime, or orange wedges for serving

In a small pitcher, combine the mineral water, juice, and stevia, and mix well. Serve over the ice, with lemon, lime, or orange wedges to squeeze in for extra flavor.

JUICE NOTE • Depending on the juice you use, you will need to adjust how much stevia you use to sweeten the spritzer. Cranberry juice is naturally more tart than cherry juice, for instance, so start with a pinch of stevia and adjust to taste.

STEVIA NOTE • A little stevia goes a very long way! Start with a pinch and add another pinch or two to taste as you go. Too much stevia will taste off.

NUTRITIONAL FACTS
Per serving: 37 calories, 0 g protein, 10 g carbohydrates, 8 g sugar, 0.2 g total fat, 4% calories from fat, 1 g fiber, 36 mg sodium

GOJI GODDESS SMOOTHIE

MAKES 2 LARGE SERVINGS

The almond extract in this recipe is optional, but it gives this smoothie a delicious cherry-like flavor. Use frozen or fresh berries in this nutrient-rich, tasty drink!

2 cups plain or vanilla low-fat nondairy milk

1 cup overripe, sliced, frozen bananas

1½ cups frozen raspberries (see Note)

¼ cup goji berries

⅛–¼ teaspoon almond extract (optional, for cherry-like flavor)

1 tablespoon coconut nectar or pure maple syrup (optional, to sweeten)

In a blender, combine the milk, bananas, raspberries, goji berries, and almond extract (if using). Puree for a few minutes to ensure that the goji berries are fully blended. Taste, and add the syrup or nectar if desired. Serve.

NOTE • You can substitute other berries, like strawberries or blueberries, for the raspberries. Frozen strawberries are more difficult to measure whole, so just roughly measure.

NUTRITIONAL FACTS
Per serving: 275 calories, 8 g protein, 59 g carbohydrates, 26 g sugar, 3 g total fat, 10% calories from fat, 16 g fiber, 110 mg sodium

DIPS AND SPREADS

ESSENTIAL HUMMUS

MAKES 8 SERVINGS (4 CUPS)

This is your hummus canvas. From here, you can tweak with more or different spices, garlic, olives, or whatever you like! One addition that is particularly tasty here is sumac. It's often used in authentic hummus recipes and adds a distinct lemony essence.

2 cans (15 ounces each) chickpeas, rinsed and drained

1 medium-large clove garlic

¼ cup freshly squeezed lemon juice

Rounded ½ teaspoon sea salt

1½–2 tablespoons tahini (see Note)

1 teaspoon ground sumac

½ teaspoon ground cumin

Several cubes of ice or a few tablespoons of cold water

In a food processor, combine the chickpeas, garlic, lemon juice, salt, tahini, sumac, and cumin. Puree, adding the ice or water as necessary to reach the desired consistency. Use just enough to get the hummus smooth while still maintaining a thick texture. Taste, and season with additional salt or spices, if desired.

NOTE • The taste and quality of tahini differs significantly by brand. Many common store-bought brands are okay, but others can be bitter and tacky. If you are able to source tahini from a specialty shop or online, try to do so. Look for an authentic tahini. Some brands to try include Al Wadi and Baron's. Some raw organic brands are also quite good, but they can be more expensive.

NUTRITIONAL FACTS
Per serving: 115 calories, 5 g protein, 17 g carbohydrates, 3 g sugar, 3 g total fat, 25% calories from fat, 5 g fiber, 367 mg sodium

SPICED SWEET POTATO HUMMUS

MAKES 4 SERVINGS

Cooked sweet potato lends creaminess and sweetness to a punchy hummus seasoned with lime juice and earthy spices.

- 1 can (15 ounces) kidney beans, rinsed (about 1¾ cups)
- 1 can (15 ounces) chickpeas, rinsed (about 1¾ cups)
- 1 cup cooked and peeled orange sweet potato (see Sweet Potato Note)
- 2 tablespoons tahini
- 1 teaspoon sea salt
- ¼ teaspoon cinnamon

- 1 medium or large clove garlic, sliced or quartered
- 4–4½ tablespoons freshly squeezed lime juice
- ½–1 teaspoon chili powder (adjust to taste; see Spice Note)
- 1–3 tablespoons water
- Fresh cilantro or parsley (optional)

In a food procesor, combine the kidney beans, chickpeas, sweet potato, tahini, salt, cinnamon, garlic, lime juice, ½ teaspoon of the chili powder, and 1 tablespoon of the water. Puree until smooth, gradually adding the remaining 2 tablespoons of water if needed to thin the hummus and scraping down the sides of the bowl as needed. Add the fresh cilantro or parsley (if using), and puree briefly to incorporate. Season with additional salt and the remaining ½ teaspoon chili powder, if desired.

SWEET POTATO NOTE • Bake more sweet potatoes than you need at a time and keep the extras refrigerated for 4 to 5 days to use in other dishes, such as salads, soups, pasta sauces, and more. Give sweet potatoes a quick wash and then bake them, whole and unpeeled, at 450°F for 40 to 60 minutes on a baking sheet lined with parchment paper. Baking time will vary based on the size of the spuds.

SPICE NOTE • Use a good quality chili powder that isn't too hot. If you aren't sure of the heat intensity, start with a lesser amount, taste, and add more if desired. You can also substitute a chipotle powder or chipotle hot sauce, to taste.

Shown in color insert pages

NUTRITIONAL FACTS
Per serving: 275 calories, 13 g protein, 43 g carbohydrates, 9 g sugar, 7 g total fat, 21% calories from fat, 11 g fiber, 914 mg sodium

FRESH SALSA

MAKES 4 SERVINGS

No store-bought salsa comes close to the flavor of fresh! It's easy to make, and it's not just for chip-dipping. Try it over cooked grains or mixed into beans or with baked tortilla chips, toasted baguette, or even an entrée.

2 cups chopped tomatoes

¼ cup minced onion or ⅓ cup chopped green onion

¼ cup minced red, yellow, or orange bell pepper

1 small jalapeño pepper, seeded and minced, wear plastic gloves when handling

1 large clove garlic, minced or grated

1 tablespoon lime juice

½ teaspoon sea salt

½ teaspoon cumin (optional)

⅛ teaspoon allspice

Freshly ground black pepper to taste

¼ cup minced cilantro (optional)

In a large bowl, combine the tomatoes, onion, bell pepper, jalapeño pepper, garlic, lime juice, salt, cumin (if using), allspice, black pepper, and cilantro (if using). Stir to combine. Taste, and add extra salt or spices as desired. Serve or refrigerate in an airtight container until ready to use (within 2 to 3 days).

NUTRITIONAL FACTS

Per serving: 27 calories, 1 g protein, 6 g carbohydrates, 3 g sugar, 0.3 g total fat, 8% calories from fat, 2 g fiber, 301 mg sodium

CHOCOLATE ORANGE DIP

MAKES 4 SERVINGS

Here's a dip to eat when your sweet tooth is calling. This treat is so nutritious you can have it any time of day! Serve with strawberries, apple or pear slices, or as a spread on small toasts.

1 cup (packed) pitted dates (see Note)

⅓ cup fresh orange juice

1 can (15 ounces) white beans, drained and rinsed

2 tablespoons almond or cashew butter (or 1½ tablespoons softened coconut butter, for nut-free)

1 teaspoon orange zest

¼ teaspoon vanilla powder or 1 teaspoon pure vanilla extract

¼ teaspoon sea salt

¼ cup cocoa powder

1–2 tablespoons coconut nectar or pure maple syrup (optional)

2 tablespoons mini chocolate chips (optional)

In a food processor, combine the dates, orange juice, white beans, nut butter, orange zest, vanilla powder or extract, and salt. Puree until smooth. Add the cocoa powder and puree again. Taste, and add the nectar or syrup to sweeten, if desired. Pulse in or garnish with the chocolate chips (if using). Serve or transfer to an airtight container and refrigerate for up to 6 days.

NOTE • If your dates are dry or hard, cover them with boiled water and let them soak for about 15 minutes. Drain off all the water, pat dry, and use as directed.

NUTRITIONAL FACTS
Per serving: 275 calories, 11 g protein, 53 g carbohydrates, 26 g sugar, 6 g total fat, 17% calories from fat, 10 g fiber, 279 mg sodium

WARM CHEESY SWEET POTATO DIP

MAKES 4 SERVINGS

This dip is lighter than many dairy-free, plant-based dips with a base of sweet potatoes—but it still has an irresistible "cheesy" quality. Serve with crusty breads or toasts, and try it in Righteous Lasagna (page 134), too!

1½ cups precooked yellow or orange sweet potatoes, skins removed (see Sweet Potato Note)

⅓ cup presoaked cashews or 2 tablespoons tahini

1 tablespoon apple cider vinegar

½ tablespoon miso

1 medium-large clove garlic

½ teaspoon sea salt

¼ teaspoon dried rosemary or 1 teaspoon fresh

¼–½ cup water (see Water Note)

Preheat the oven to 375°F. In a blender, combine the potatoes, cashews or tahini, vinegar, miso, garlic, salt, rosemary, and water. Puree until very smooth. Transfer to a small baking dish. Bake for 25 to 30 minutes, until golden in spots.

SWEET POTATO NOTE • It's great to bake sweet potatoes whole. Line a baking sheet with parchment paper. Give the spuds a quick wash, then put them on the baking sheet and bake at 450°F for 40 to 60 minutes, until tender. (Baking time will depend on the size of the sweet potatoes.)

WATER NOTE • If using orange sweet potatoes, they need a little less water to puree. Try using ¼ to ⅓ cup.

NUTRITIONAL FACTS
Per serving: 125 calories, 4 g protein, 18 g carbohydrates, 5 g sugar, 5 g total fat, 33% calories from fat, 3 g fiber, 399 mg sodium

GREEN-WITH-ENVY GUACAMOLE

MAKES 4 SERVINGS

Boost traditional guacamole with the green goodness of baby spinach and green chickpeas.

1½ cups packed roughly chopped or sliced ripe avocado

1 cup packed baby spinach

½ cup green chickpeas (frozen), edamame (frozen), or white beans (see Note)

¾ teaspoon sea salt

3 tablespoons lime or lemon juice

¼–⅓ cup water

½ teaspoon coconut nectar or pure maple syrup (optional)

In a food processor or high-speed blender, combine the avocado, spinach, chickpeas, salt, lime or lemon juice, and ¼ cup of the water. Puree until smooth. Add the remaining water if needed to thin or smoothly puree. Taste, and add the nectar or syrup to balance the flavor, if desired.

NOTE • The green chickpeas or edamame can be used frozen if you're using a high-powered blender. If you're using a standard blender, thaw them and then puree.

Shown in color insert pages

NUTRITIONAL FACTS
Per serving: 132 calories, 3 g protein, 12 g carbohydrates, 2 g sugar, 9 g total fat, 59% calories from fat, 6 g fiber, 453 mg sodium

AVOCADO HUMMUS

MAKES 8 SERVINGS (ABOUT 4 CUPS)

A touch of avocado adds richness, and white beans lend an extra-creamy texture to this twist on hummus. A must-make!

2   cans (15 ounces each) white beans, rinsed and drained

¼   cup lime juice

2–3   tablespoons fresh parsley leaves

¾   teaspoon sea salt

1   large clove garlic

¼   teaspoon ground cumin

Freshly ground black pepper or lemon pepper to taste

1   cup cubed avocado (1½–2 avocados, depending on size)

In a food processor, combine the beans, lime juice, parsley, salt, garlic, cumin, and pepper, and puree until very smooth. Add the avocado and puree to combine. Season with additional salt and pepper to taste. Serve.

NUTRITIONAL FACTS

Per serving: 135 calories, 8 g protein, 21 g carbohydrates, 1 g sugar, 3 g total fat, 20% calories from fat, 6 g fiber, 336 mg sodium

GREEN CHICKPEA HUMMUS

MAKES 6 SERVINGS (ABOUT 3 CUPS)

It's easy eating green with this fresh take on hummus! Green chickpeas step in for their cooked legume counterpart in this tangy, flavorful dip!

2 cups frozen green chickpeas (see Chickpeas Note)

1 can (15 ounces) white beans, rinsed and drained

¼ cup lemon juice

1 large clove garlic (or more to taste)

⅓ cup fresh basil leaves

⅓ cup fresh parsley leaves

1 tablespoon tahini

1 teaspoon sea salt

½ teaspoon ground cumin

1–2 tablespoons water (optional)

½ teaspoon lemon zest (optional)

Add the chickpeas to a pot of boiling water and cook for just a minute to bring out their vibrant green color. Remove, run under cold water to stop the cooking process, and drain. In a food processor (see Food Processor Note), combine the chickpeas, beans, lemon juice, garlic, basil, parsley, tahini, salt, and cumin. Puree until smooth, scraping down the bowl as needed. Add the water if desired to thin or help the pureeing process. Add the lemon zest, if desired, and season to taste. Serve.

CHICKPEAS NOTE • If you cannot find green chickpeas, use a combination of green peas and edamame (half of each, preferably).

FOOD PROCESSOR NOTE • A high-speed blender will give you a smoother consistency; a food processor will give you more texture.

NUTRITIONAL FACTS
Per serving: 176 calories, 10 g protein, 29 g carbohydrates, 3 g sugar, 3 g total fat, 14% calories from fat, 8 g fiber, 477 mg sodium

CREAMY ROASTED RED PEPPER DIP

MAKES 7 SERVINGS (ABOUT 1¾ CUPS)

This red pepper dip is creamy and has a few extra flavor notes beyond the peppers themselves. The basil is optional, but it adds a nice flavor. This dip is great with pita breads or tortilla chips but is also dynamite spread on sandwiches, added to wraps, or tossed into pasta!

2 large red peppers (see Roasted Peppers Note)	½ tablespoon chickpea miso (or other mild-flavored miso)
Pinch + ½ teaspoon sea salt	1 small clove garlic (or more to taste)
½ cup precooked white potato, skin removed, cubed or roughly chopped (not packed to measure)	1–2 tablespoons water (optional)
	¼–½ teaspoon pure maple syrup (optional; see Maple Syrup Note)
1 tablespoon red wine vinegar	¼ cup loosely packed fresh basil leaves (optional)
1 tablespoon tahini	
1 tablespoon nutritional yeast	

Preheat the oven to broil. Line a baking sheet with parchment paper.

Core the peppers, remove the seeds, and cut the pepper flesh into 3 or 4 large pieces. Place them on the prepared baking sheet, skin sides up. Sprinkle with a pinch of salt. Place in the oven for 12 to 15 minutes, or until the peppers are well charred and blistered. Remove from the oven and transfer to a glass bowl that is deep enough to hold the peppers below its top edge. Cover the bowl with plastic wrap and let sit for 20 to 30 minutes. Remove the skins (they should slip off easily) and discard.

In a blender, combine the peppers with the potato, vinegar, tahini, yeast, miso, garlic, and the remaining ½ teaspoon of salt. Puree until smooth. Depending on the liquid in the peppers and how powerful your blender is, you may need to thin slightly with the water. Add 1 tablespoon at a time, puree, and check the consistency. Taste and decide if you'd like to add the syrup. Add the basil (if using), and puree. Season to taste. Serve at room temperature, or place in a heat-proof dish and heat in the oven until warmed through.

ROASTED PEPPERS NOTE • If you want to use jarred roasted red peppers, that's fine. Drain well and measure 1¼ to 1½ cups.

MAPLE SYRUP NOTE • The sweetness of bell peppers can vary based on the time of year, where you buy them, etc. For that reason, you may want to add the maple syrup.

IDEA: Try using as a pasta sauce!

Shown in color insert pages

NUTRITIONAL FACTS
Per serving: 42 calories, 2 g protein, 6 g carbohydrates, 2 g sugar, 1 g total fat, 28% calories from fat, 1 g fiber, 259 mg sodium

LENTIL BABA GHANOUSH

MAKES 4 SERVINGS (ABOUT 2 CUPS)

Here's a version of baba ghanoush that thinks beyond the traditional eggplant. The flavors are similar to the traditional version, yet it's also heartier because of the addition of brown lentils.

2 cups cooked brown lentils	½ teaspoon lemon zest
1½ tablespoons chopped fresh oregano leaves	2 tablespoons tahini
1 large clove garlic	3½–4 tablespoons lemon juice
½ teaspoon sea salt	1–4 tablespoons water (as needed to smooth, see Note)
Rounded ¼ teaspoon smoked paprika	Drizzle of tamari (optional)

In a food processor, combine the lentils, oregano, garlic, salt, paprika, lemon zest, tahini, and 3½ tablespoons of the lemon juice. Puree until smooth, adding the water as needed, 1 tablespoon at a time. Taste, and add the remaining ½ tablespoon lemon juice, if desired. Serve, adding a drizzle of tamari (if using).

NOTE • Depending on the moisture in the cooked lentils, you may not need the water. After pureeing, if the mixture is dry, add the water to smooth.

NUTRITIONAL FACTS
Per serving: 165 calories, 10 g protein, 23 g carbohydrates, 1 g sugar, 5 g total fat, 23% calories from fat, 7 g fiber, 307 mg sodium

ASIAN-FUSION HUMMUS

MAKES 8 SERVINGS (ABOUT 4 CUPS)

Hummus takes on a slightly exotic twist with the addition of lime and orange juices, plus a hit of ginger. Delicious!

4 cups cooked chickpeas (rinse and drain if using canned)

2 tablespoons orange juice

3 tablespoons peanut butter or tahini

1 medium-large clove garlic, sliced

1 tablespoon grated fresh ginger

1 pitted date

3 tablespoons tamari

¼–⅓ cup freshly squeezed lime juice

2–4 tablespoons water

Sea salt to taste

⅛ teaspoon crushed red-pepper flakes (optional)

In a food processor, combine the chickpeas, orange juice, peanut butter or tahini, garlic, ginger, date, tamari, ¼ cup of the lime juice, and 2 tablespoons of the water. Puree until very smooth. Taste, and add the remaining lime juice for more tang, if you like, and the additional 2 tablespoons of water, if needed to achieve a smoother texture. Puree until well combined. Add salt to taste and the red-pepper flakes (if using).

NUTRITIONAL FACTS
Per serving: 182 calories, 9 g protein, 26 g carbohydrates, 6 g sugar, 5 g total fat, 24% calories from fat, 7 g fiber, 555 mg sodium

SMOKY RED DIP

MAKES 7 SERVINGS (ABOUT 3½ CUPS)

While the color is more pink than red, this dip combines roasted red peppers with red lentils and a robust smoky essence. Divine!

- 3 cups cooked red lentils (see Lentils Note)
- 1 cup roasted red peppers (see Red Peppers Note)
- 1½–2 tablespoons tahini
- 1½ tablespoons red wine vinegar
- 1 tablespoon nutritional yeast
- ¾ teaspoon sea salt
- ½ teaspoon smoked paprika or ¼ teaspoon chipotle powder (or both!)
- ½–1 tablespoon chickpea miso, or other mild-flavored miso (see Miso Note)
- 1–2 medium-large cloves garlic

In a food processor, combine the lentils, peppers, tahini, vinegar, yeast, salt, paprika or chipotle powder, ½ tablespoon of the miso, and 1 clove of the garlic. Puree until very smooth. Taste, and add the additional ½ tablespoon miso if desired, and the additional clove of garlic, if you want more garlic kick. Serve, or refrigerate to serve later. The dip will thicken after chilling.

LENTILS NOTE • If cooking from dry, this is roughly 1 cup of dry red lentils.

RED PEPPERS NOTE • If roasting yourself, 2 medium red bell peppers will yield about 1 cup. (See Creamy Roasted Red Pepper Dip on page 70.)

MISO NOTE • Chickpea miso has a fabulous mellow flavor. If you cannot find it, however, feel free to substitute another mellow miso, such as brown rice miso.

NUTRITIONAL FACTS
Per serving: 132 calories, 9 g protein, 20 g carbohydrates, 1 g sugar, 2 g total fat, 14% calories from fat, 6 g fiber, 303 mg sodium

SALSA MAKEOVER

MAKES 5 SERVINGS (ABOUT 2½ CUPS)

While fresh salsa has the best flavor, you can elevate the taste of store-bought salsa with a few additions from your kitchen.

1   cup store-bought fresh or jarred salsa

⅔   cup small cubes ripe avocado (about 1 avocado)

½   cup diced red pepper

½   cup frozen corn kernels, thawed in a bowl of boiled water

½   tablespoon lime juice

Few tablespoons chopped fresh cilantro or fresh parsley (optional)

Sea salt

Freshly ground pepper to taste (optional)

In a large bowl, combine the salsa, avocado, red pepper, corn, lime juice, and cilantro or parsley (if using). Mix together. Season to taste with salt and pepper, if using.

NUTRITIONAL FACTS

Per serving: 78 calories, 2 g protein, 10 g carbohydrates, 3 g sugar, 4 g total fat, 48% calories from fat, 3 g fiber, 368 mg sodium

IRRESISTIBLE WHITE BEAN DIP

MAKES 4 SERVINGS (ABOUT 2 CUPS)

This recipe is ready in just minutes. The combination of miso, black salt, and nutritional yeast makes it irresistible!

1 can (15 ounces) white beans, rinsed and drained

2 tablespoons lemon juice

2 teaspoons miso

Scant ½ teaspoon sea salt

¼ teaspoon black salt

1 tablespoon tahini

1 tablespoon nutritional yeast

1 clove garlic (or to taste)

¼–½ teaspoon pure maple syrup (optional)

1–1½ tablespoons water

In a small food processor or high-powered blender, combine the beans, lemon juice, miso, sea salt, black salt, tahini, yeast, garlic, syrup (if using), and 1 table-spoon of the water. Puree, adding the additional ½ tablespoon water if needed. (Just don't add too much; the dip should be thick.) Taste, and season with extra lemon, salt, or garlic, if desired.

NUTRITIONAL FACTS

Per serving: 139 calories, 9 g protein, 21 g carbohydrates, 1 g sugar, 3 g total fat, 16% calories from fat, 6 g fiber, 638 mg sodium

SAUCES, DRESSINGS, SALADS, AND SANDWICHES

FUSS-FREE GRAVY

MAKES ABOUT 5 SERVINGS (1¾ CUPS)

This gravy is so easy to make. Whisk, bubble, and pour!

3 tablespoons millet flour (see Note)

½ tablespoon red wine vinegar

1 tablespoon tahini

1 tablespoon tomato paste

1 teaspoon garlic powder

½ teaspoon onion powder

2½–3 tablespoons tamari

1–2 tablespoons nutritional yeast (to taste)

1½ cups water

2 teaspoons fresh chopped rosemary or ½ teaspoon dried

1–1½ teaspoons coconut nectar or pure maple syrup

Sea salt to taste

Freshly ground black pepper to taste

In a small saucepan over medium heat, combine the flour, vinegar, tahini, tomato paste, garlic powder, onion powder, 2½ tablespoons of the tamari, and 1 table-spoon of the nutritional yeast. Whisk for a couple of minutes. Add a few table-spoons of the water and continue to whisk. The mixture will be very thick, but keep working it to cook out the raw flavor of the flour. Add about ¼ cup more water and continuously whisk and heat the mixture. Slowly add the remaining water, whisking as you go. Once all the water has been added and the mixture is well combined, add the rosemary and 1 teaspoon of the nectar or syrup, and bring to a boil. Reduce the heat to low and simmer for 7 to 8 minutes. If the mixture becomes too thick, add a touch more water to thin, whisking it in. Taste, and add the remaining ½ tablespoon tamari, 1 table-spoon nutritional yeast, ½ teaspoon nectar or syrup, and salt or pepper, if desired. Serve.

NOTE • You can substitute another flour here, such as spelt or whole wheat pastry flour. Millet flour is especially nice to use because it doesn't clump the way gluten-based flours can. But, if you whisk well at the beginning while adding the water, any flour can be used.

NUTRITIONAL FACTS
Per ⅓-cup serving: 53 calories, 3 g protein, 7 g carbohydrates, 1 g sugar, 2 g total fat, 30% calories from fat, 1 g fiber, 506 mg sodium

LIGHTENED TAHINI SAUCE

MAKES 8 SERVINGS (ABOUT 1 CUP)

This tahini sauce is light and delicious.

⅓ cup tahini

⅓ cup unsweetened applesauce

3 tablespoons lemon juice

2 tablespoons tamari

1–2 teaspoons coconut nectar (optional)

2–4 tablespoons water

Sea salt

Freshly ground black pepper

In a blender (or using an immersion blender and a deep cup), combine the tahini, applesauce, lemon juice, tamari, nectar (if using), 2 tablespoons of the water, and salt and pepper to taste. Puree until smooth. Add the additional 1 to 2 tablespoons water if desired to thin the sauce. Season to taste, and serve.

Shown in color insert pages

NUTRITIONAL FACTS

Per 2-tablespoon serving: 68 calories, 2 g protein, 4 g carbohydrates, 1 g sugar, 5 g total fat, 67% calories from fat, 1 g fiber, 559 mg sodium

BALSAMIC DRIZZLE

MAKES 5 SERVINGS (ABOUT ⅓ CUP)

Serve this balsamic reduction drizzled over Miso Rice Patties (page 144) or over just about any other dish that you'd like to add a good pop of flavor to! The smell of vinegar can be strong while simmering, so open a window in your kitchen if you can.

½ cup balsamic vinegar   Pinch or two of sea salt
2 tablespoons coconut nectar

In a saucepan over medium-high heat, combine the vinegar, coconut nectar, and salt. Bring the mixture to a boil, then reduce the heat to medium-low. Let the mixture gently boil for 25 to 30 minutes, or until it has thickened and reduced in volume. If you'd like it thicker, let it cook for a few additional minutes. Remove from the heat and let it cool. (It will thicken a little more with cooling.) Leftovers can be stored in a jar or bottle in the fridge.

IDEA: If you love balsamic reductions, make a double batch of this so you can store the extra in the fridge.

NUTRITIONAL FACTS
Per 1-tablespoon serving: 40 calories, 0 g protein, 9 g carbohydrates, 8 g sugar, 0 g total fat, 0% calories from fat, 0 g fiber, 62 mg sodium

LIME ZINGER DRESSING

MAKES 4 SERVINGS (ABOUT ½ CUP)

Love the punch of fresh lime juice? Try this dressing on a dinner salad, or even on cooked grains or lentils.

¼ cup freshly squeezed lime juice

3 tablespoons coconut nectar

½ tablespoon ground chia seeds

½ tablespoon Dijon mustard

½ teaspoon ground cumin

¼ teaspoon cinnamon

Pinch of allspice

½ teaspoon sea salt

Freshly ground black pepper to taste

1 tablespoon water (optional)

In a blender, combine the lime juice, nectar, chia seeds, mustard, cumin, cinnamon, allspice, salt, and pepper. Puree until smooth. Add the water if desired to thin. Transfer to a jar or other airtight container and refrigerate for up to a week.

NOTE • This dressing will thicken with refrigeration. To thin, simply whisk in another 1 to 2 teaspoons of water.

NUTRITIONAL FACTS
Per 2-tablespoon serving: 52 calories, 0 g protein, 12 g carbohydrates, 9 g sugar, 1 g total fat, 9% calories from fat, 1 g fiber, 340 mg sodium

GREEN GODDESS DRESSING

MAKES 5 SERVINGS (ABOUT ⅔ CUP)

Fresh herbs like parsley and basil are delicious and healthful. You'll make the most of them in this creamy, aromatic dressing.

⅓ cup cooked white beans (such as cannellini or navy) or ¼ cup soaked cashews

¼–⅓ cup water if using white beans, or ⅓–½ cup if using cashews

⅓ cup loosely packed fresh basil leaves

¼ cup loosely packed fresh parsley leaves

1–1½ tablespoons tahini (use full 1½ tablespoons tahini with white beans or ½–1 tablespoon with cashews; see Note)

2½ tablespoons freshly squeezed lemon juice

2 teaspoons pure maple syrup

½ teaspoon Dijon mustard

1 very small clove garlic

½ teaspoon sea salt

Freshly ground black pepper to taste (optional)

In a blender, combine the beans, water, basil, parsley, tahini, lemon juice, syrup, mustard, garlic, salt, and pepper (if using). Puree until smooth. Season to taste with additional salt and pepper, and serve or refrigerate. Keeps for 3 to 4 days in the fridge.

NOTE • The cashew version is naturally creamy. For a creamier version of the white bean version, use the full amount of tahini. If you like, add a handful of baby spinach to the blend for an extra boost of greens!

NUTRITIONAL FACTS
Per 2-tablespoon serving: 42 calories, 2 g protein, 6 g carbohydrates, 2 g sugar, 2 g total fat, 32% calories from fat, 1 g fiber, 237 mg sodium

MANGO-HEMP DRESSING

MAKES 8 SERVINGS (ABOUT 1 CUP)

This dressing will bring new life to salads!

¾ cup mango chunks, fresh or frozen

2 tablespoons hemp seeds

2 tablespoons freshly squeezed lime juice or red wine vinegar

½ tablespoon chopped shallots or 1 tablespoon of the whitish portion of a green onion

½ teaspoon Dijon mustard

½ teaspoon sea salt

Freshly ground black pepper to taste

¼ cup + 2–3 teaspoons water (optional)

1–2 tablespoons coconut nectar or pure maple syrup

In a blender, combine the mango, hemp, lime juice or vinegar, shallots or green onion, mustard, salt, pepper, ¼ cup of the water, and 1 tablespoon of the nectar or syrup. Puree until very smooth. Taste, and add the remaining 2 to 3 tablespoons water to thin (if desired) and the remaining 1 tablespoon nectar or syrup, to taste.

IDEA: If you'd like to pair this dressing with some spicy foods or add an extra punch of flavor, try adding 1 to 2 tablespoons of chopped cilantro or basil while pureeing.

NUTRITIONAL FACTS
Per 2-tablespoon serving: 31 calories, 1 g protein, 5 g carbohydrates, 4 g sugar, 1 g total fat, 28% calories from fat, 1 g fiber, 155 mg sodium

PUNCHY MUSTARD VINAIGRETTE

MAKES 6 SERVINGS (ABOUT ¾ CUP)

If you love a good mustardy dressing, this is the one for you! Bonus: It's ridiculously easy to make.

- ¼ cup apple cider vinegar or rice vinegar
- 2 tablespoons tamari
- 1½ tablespoons yellow or Dijon mustard
- 2½ tablespoons coconut nectar or pure maple syrup

- ½ tablespoon ground chia
  Freshly ground black pepper to taste
- ⅛ teaspoon sea salt

In a blender, combine the vinegar, tamari, mustard, nectar or syrup, chia, pepper, and salt. Puree until fully incorporated. Taste, and add extra mustard if you love it! Season to taste with additional salt and pepper, if desired. Serve immediately or refrigerate. Dressing will keep for at least a week in the fridge.

NUTRITIONAL FACTS
Per 2-tablespoon serving: 33 calories, 1 g protein, 7 g carbohydrates, 5 g sugar, 0.4 g total fat, 11% calories from fat, 1 g fiber, 428 mg sodium

DREAMY CAESAR DRESSING

MAKES 12 SERVINGS (ABOUT 1½ CUPS)

This dressing is lusciously creamy, without a drop of dairy or oil!

¼–⅓ cup soaked almonds or cashews

½ cup cooked red or yellow potato, skins removed (see Note)

2 tablespoons freshly squeezed lemon juice

1½ tablespoons red wine vinegar

1 medium or large clove garlic, chopped (adjust to taste)

1 tablespoon chickpea miso (or other mild-flavored miso)

2 teaspoons Dijon mustard

½ teaspoon sea salt

Freshly ground black pepper to taste

1 teaspoon pure maple syrup

¾ cup plain low-fat nondairy milk

2–3 tablespoons water or nondairy milk (optional)

In a blender, combine the nuts, potato, lemon juice, vinegar, garlic, miso, mustard, salt, pepper, syrup, and milk. Puree until very smooth. Add the water or additional milk to thin the dressing, if desired. (It will thicken after refrigeration.)

NOTE • Advance cooking of staples like potatoes helps with quick prep of recipes like this one. Simply bake or steam several potatoes until fully softened. Refrigerate for up to 6 days, until ready to use.

Shown in color insert pages

NUTRITIONAL FACTS
Per 2-tablespoon serving: 34 calories, 1 g protein, 4 g carbohydrates, 1 g sugar, 2 g total fat, 42% calories from fat, 1 g fiber, 177 mg sodium

AVOCADO BASIL DRESSING

MAKES 6 SERVINGS (ABOUT ¾ CUP)

This thick, creamy dressing is irresistible on salads, cooked beans, whole grains, or baked potatoes.

¾ cup cubed ripe avocado (about 1 medium avocado)

1½ tablespoons freshly squeezed lemon juice

¼ cup loosely packed fresh basil leaves

Rounded ¼ teaspoon sea salt

Freshly ground black pepper to taste

½ cup + 1–2 tablespoons water

1–1½ teaspoons coconut nectar or pure maple syrup

In a blender, combine the avocado, lemon juice, basil, salt, pepper, ½ cup of the water, and 1 teaspoon of the nectar or syrup. Puree until very smooth. Add the additional 1 to 2 tablespoons water to thin to the desired consistency and the additional ½ teaspoon of nectar or syrup, if desired. Season with additional salt and pepper to taste.

NUTRITIONAL FACTS

Per 2-tablespoon serving: 41 calories, 0 g protein, 4 g carbohydrates, 2 g sugar, 3 g total fat, 59% calories from fat, 1 g fiber, 149 mg sodium

MOROCCAN SALAD DRESSING

MAKES 5 SERVINGS (ABOUT ⅔ CUP)

Use this dressing for a superbly satisfying Moroccan Bean Salad! Also try over steamed greens and salads.

¼ cup lemon juice	1 very small clove garlic
¼ cup water	¼ teaspoon paprika
1 tablespoon tahini	½ teaspoon ground cumin
1½ tablespoons pure maple syrup	½ teaspoon cinnamon
2 teaspoons roughly chopped fresh ginger	½ teaspoon sea salt

In a blender, combine the lemon juice, water, tahini, syrup, ginger, garlic, paprika, cumin, cinnamon, and salt. Puree until smooth.

Shown in color insert pages

NUTRITIONAL FACTS

Per 2-tablespoon serving: 36 calories, 1 g protein, 6 g carbohydrates, 4 g sugar, 2 g total fat, 37% calories from fat, 1 g fiber, 227 mg sodium

MOROCCAN BEAN SALAD

MAKES 4 SERVINGS

Here's a party-worthy salad! It's flavorful, chunky, satisfying, and easy to make.

1   can (15 ounces) chickpeas, rinsed and drained

1   can (15 ounces) black beans, rinsed and drained (or 1½ cups cooked grain, such as brown rice or quinoa)

1   cup diced red pepper

½   cup diced raw zucchini (can substitute cucumber)

⅓   cup chopped dried apricots

⅓   cup green onions

2   cups roughly chopped baby spinach

½   cup Moroccan Salad Dressing

    Sea salt to taste

    Freshly ground black pepper to taste

In a large bowl, combine the chickpeas, beans, red pepper, zucchini, apricots, onions, and spinach. Toss to combine. Add the dressing, and toss to coat. Taste, add more dressing if desired, and season to taste with salt and black pepper. Serve, or cover and refrigerate for several hours.

Shown in color insert pages

NUTRITIONAL FACTS

Per serving: 278 calories, 13 g protein, 50 g carbohydrates, 15 g sugar, 4 g total fat, 13% calories from fat, 15 g fiber, 527 mg sodium

POWER LUNCH BOWL

MAKES 2 SERVINGS

Once you start making salad bowls, you'll fall in love with them! Here's one to get you started. Feel free to substitute other vegetables, beans, or grains as you desire.

2   cups cooked quinoa or brown rice (cold or warm, as desired)

3   cups chopped kale leaves (raw or steamed; see Note) or baby spinach leaves

2   cups cubed cooked sweet potato

1   can (15 ounces) black beans, rinsed and drained

1   cup chopped bell pepper

¼   cup Mango-Hemp Dressing (page 86) or Dreamy Caesar Dressing (page 88)

In 2 bowls, arrange approximately equal amounts of the quinoa or rice, kale or spinach, sweet potato, black beans, and bell pepper. Drizzle on the dressing of your choice.

NOTE • If using raw kale, it's useful to break it down slightly by massaging it. After tearing the leaves from the stalks, sprinkle the leaves with salt and use your hands to rub and "massage" them for a minute or two. The color will change to a brighter green and the leaves will soften. Once at this stage, chop the leaves for the salad bowl. Alternatively, you can steam the kale for just a minute to soften, and then chop it.

NUTRITIONAL FACTS

Per serving (with Mango-Hemp Dressing): 644 calories, 27 g protein, 124 g carbohydrates, 22 g sugar, 6 g total fat, 9% calories from fat, 28 g fiber, 516 mg sodium

GREEK RICE SALAD

MAKES 4 SERVINGS

If you love the flavors in a traditional Greek salad, this rice salad will become a favorite!

3 tablespoons fresh lemon juice

1½ tablespoons coconut nectar or pure maple syrup

1 tablespoon red wine vinegar

1 teaspoon sea salt

1 teaspoon Dijon mustard

¼ teaspoon allspice

½–1 teaspoon grated fresh garlic
Freshly ground black pepper to taste (optional)

4 cups cooked brown rice

1 cup chopped cucumber (seeds removed, if you prefer)

1 cup sliced grape or cherry tomatoes or chopped tomatoes (can substitute chopped red pepper)

½ cup sliced kalamata olives

½ tablespoon chopped fresh oregano

2 tablespoons chopped fresh dill

In a large bowl, whisk together the lemon juice, nectar or syrup, vinegar, salt, mustard, allspice, garlic, and pepper (if using). Add the rice, cucumber, tomatoes, olives, oregano, and dill, and stir to combine. Taste, and add extra salt or lemon juice, if desired. Serve as a side or as a hearty lunch over greens.

SERVING IDEAS: Try substituting 1 cup of the cooked rice with 1 cup of cooked beans, such as chickpeas or kidney beans. For a greens boost, reduce the tomatoes to ½ cup (or omit altogether) and add 1 to 2 cups of chopped baby spinach leaves.

NUTRITIONAL FACTS
Per serving: 306 calories, 6 g protein, 62 g carbohydrates, 7 g sugar, 4 g total fat, 11% calories from fat, 5 g fiber, 751 mg sodium

RAINBOW QUINOA SALAD

MAKES 3 SERVINGS

Quinoa with colorful, crunchy veggies and a tangy-sweet dressing makes it easy to "eat the rainbow"!

Dressing

- 3½ tablespoons orange juice
- 1 tablespoon apple cider vinegar
- 1 tablespoon pure maple syrup
- 1½ teaspoons yellow mustard
  Couple pinches of cloves
  Rounded ½ teaspoon sea salt
  Freshly ground black pepper to taste

Salad

- 2 cups cooked quinoa, cooled
- ½ cup corn kernels
- ½ cup diced apple tossed in ½ teaspoon lemon juice
- ¼ cup diced red pepper
- ¼ cup sliced green onions or chives
- 1 can (15 ounces) black beans, rinsed and drained
  Sea salt to taste
  Freshly ground black pepper to taste

To make the dressing: In a large bowl, whisk together the orange juice, vinegar, syrup, mustard, cloves, salt, and pepper.

To make the salad: Add the quinoa, corn, apple, red pepper, green onion or chives, and black beans, and stir to combine well. Season with the salt and black pepper to taste. Serve, or store in an airtight container in the fridge.

Shown in color insert pages

NUTRITIONAL FACTS

Per serving: 355 calories, 15 g protein, 68 g carbohydrates, 12 g sugar, 4 g total fat, 9% calories from fat, 15 g fiber, 955 mg sodium

WINTER FRUIT SALAD

MAKES 4 SERVINGS

This salad is made with fruits that are easy to find through fall and winter, and even into spring.

3 cups cored, chopped apples (peels optional)

3 cups cored, chopped pears (peels optional)

2 cups peeled, cubed oranges, mandarins, or grapefruit

1 cup ripe sliced bananas

1½ tablespoons freshly squeezed orange juice

⅛ teaspoon cinnamon

In a large bowl, combine the apples, pears, citrus, bananas, orange juice, and cinnamon. Toss gently to combine.

Shown in color insert pages

NUTRITIONAL FACTS

Per serving: 196 calories, 2 g protein, 51 g carbohydrates, 35 g sugar, 1 g total fat, 2% calories from fat, 9 g fiber, 3 mg sodium

SUMMER FRUIT SALAD

MAKES 4 SERVINGS

When summer produce is in full swing, this salad is nature's candy.

3 cups hulled and halved (or quartered, if large) strawberries (see Note)

2 cups blueberries

2 cups cubed pitted peaches or nectarines

2 cups cubed pitted plums

1½ tablespoons orange juice (or ½ tablespoon lemon juice)

In a large bowl, combine the strawberries, blueberries, peaches or nectarines, and plums. Add the orange juice and toss gently to combine.

NOTE • Feel free to switch up the combination of berries to include raspberries and/or blackberries.

Shown in color insert pages

NUTRITIONAL FACTS
Per serving: 152 calories, 3 g protein, 38 g carbohydrates, 29 g sugar, 1 g total fat, 6% calories from fat, 6 g fiber, 2 mg sodium

TU-NO SALAD

MAKES 2 SERVINGS

Chickpeas are the secret ingredient in this healthful, tasty salad.

1   can (15 ounces) chickpeas, rinsed and drained

1   tablespoon tahini

2   tablespoons water

1   tablespoon red wine vinegar (can substitute apple cider vinegar)

1   tablespoon chickpea miso (or other mild-flavored miso)

1   teaspoon vegan Worcestershire sauce (optional)

½   teaspoon Dijon mustard

½   teaspoon coconut nectar

2   tablespoons minced celery (see Note)

2   tablespoons minced cucumber

2   tablespoons minced apple

⅛   teaspoon sea salt
    Freshly ground black pepper to taste

In a small food processor, pulse the chickpeas until fairly crumbly but not finely ground. (Alternatively, you can mash by hand.) In a large bowl, combine the chickpeas, tahini, water, vinegar, miso, Worcestershire sauce, mustard, nectar, celery, cucumber, apple, and salt. Mix together well. Season with additional salt and pepper to taste, and serve!

NOTE • You can substitute minced bell pepper or just 1 tablespoon of minced green onions for the celery, cucumber, or apple.

SERVING SUGGESTIONS: Serve in pitas or, more traditionally, sandwiched between slices of whole grain bread. Other ideas include spooning into romaine hearts (for lettuce "cups") or using as a filling in a whole grain tortilla wrap.

NUTRITIONAL FACTS
Per serving: 264 calories, 12 g protein, 37 g carbohydrates, 8 g sugar, 8 g total fat, 27% calories from fat, 10 g fiber, 800 mg sodium

CHIPOTLE-KISSED CORN SALAD

MAKES 4 SERVINGS

This salad comes together in a snap and is wonderful for potlucks and summer barbecues.

2½ cups corn kernels	¼ cup chopped chives
1 can (15 ounces) white beans, rinsed and drained	½–1 teaspoon chipotle hot sauce (see Note)
1 cup chopped red pepper	¼–⅓ cup Lime Zinger Dressing (page 84)
¼ cup diced cucumber	

In a salad bowl, combine the corn, beans, pepper, cucumber, and chives, and mix thoroughly. Add ½ teaspoon of the hot sauce and ¼ cup of the dressing. Taste, and add the remaining hot sauce or dressing to taste. Serve, or store in an air-tight container in the refrigerator for up to 3 days.

NOTE • The heat of these sauces can vary, so start with about ½ teaspoon, and use more if you like.

NUTRITIONAL FACTS
Per serving: 221 calories, 10 g protein, 46 g carbohydrates, 10 g sugar, 1 g total fat, 5% calories from fat, 8 g fiber, 302 mg sodium

CHEESY CROUTONS

MAKES 4 SERVINGS

Bye-bye oily, store-bought croutons—hello cheesy croutons!

1½ tablespoons aquafaba (see Note)

1½ tablespoons nutritional yeast

⅛ teaspoon garlic powder

¼ teaspoon sea salt

3 cups 1" cubes sprouted grain bread

Preheat the oven to 375°F. Line a baking sheet with parchment paper.

In a large bowl, whisk together the aquafaba, yeast, garlic powder, and salt. Add the bread and toss it in the mixture, using your fingers. Transfer the cubes to the prepared baking sheet. Bake for about 12 minutes, tossing a couple of times. If the croutons look golden and are becoming crisp, turn off the heat and let sit in the warm oven for another few minutes to crisp up. If not, bake for another minute or two, checking on them frequently, as they can go from golden to burned very quickly. Let cool on the pan, then use immediately.

NOTE • "Aquafaba" simply means "bean water." It is the liquid drained from a can of beans, preferably white beans or chickpeas.

NUTRITIONAL FACTS

Per serving: 90 calories, 4 g protein, 16 g carbohydrates, 1 g sugar, 1 g total fat, 11% calories from fat, 2 g fiber, 327 mg sodium

BRAVO-CADO PASTA SALAD

MAKES 4 SERVINGS

Tender pasta noodles are tossed with a luscious avocado-based dressing in this fresh take on pasta.

6   cups cooked cut pasta (such as rotini or penne), cooled

½   cup sliced cherry tomatoes

½   cup chopped bell pepper

½   cup halved black olives

½   cup chopped dry-pack sun-dried tomatoes

2   tablespoons sliced chives

¼   cup julienned fresh basil leaves

½   tablespoon freshly squeezed lemon juice or red wine vinegar

⅛   teaspoon sea salt

Freshly ground black pepper to taste

1   batch Avocado Basil Dressing (page 89)

½   avocado, cut into small cubes (optional)

In a large bowl, combine the pasta, cherry tomatoes, bell pepper, olives, sun-dried tomatoes, chives, basil, lemon juice or vinegar, salt, black pepper, dressing, and cubed avocado, if using. Gently toss, coating the pasta well with the dressing. Season to taste and serve.

NUTRITIONAL FACTS
Per serving: 442 calories, 14 g protein, 78 g carbohydrates, 8 g sugar, 9 g total fat, 16% calories from fat, 8 g fiber, 577 mg sodium

QUINOA KALE CAESAR

MAKES 3 SERVINGS

Kale and quinoa pair up for this fresh and hearty twist on a classic Caesar.

2 cups cooked quinoa	¼ teaspoon sea salt
3–4 cups chopped kale leaves (tear leaves from stem first, then chop)	Freshly ground black pepper to taste
½–⅔ cup Dreamy Caesar Dressing (page 88)	1½ cups Cheesy Croutons (page 99)
1 tablespoon lemon juice	

In a large bowl, combine the quinoa, kale, dressing, lemon juice, salt, and pepper. Toss to combine. Season with extra lemon juice, salt, or pepper to taste. Add the croutons just before serving so they stay crunchy.

NUTRITIONAL FACTS

Per serving: 266 calories, 11 g protein, 44 g carbohydrates, 5 g sugar, 6 g total fat, 19% calories from fat, 6 g fiber, 662 mg sodium

ITALIAN BEAN SALAD

MAKES 4 SERVINGS

Every bite offers a different flavor. This is a great dish for parties and potlucks.

- 2 tablespoons lemon juice
- 1 tablespoon red wine vinegar
- 1 tablespoon pure maple syrup
- 1½ teaspoons Dijon mustard
  Rounded ¼ teaspoon sea salt
- ½ teaspoon dried oregano
- ¼ teaspoon garlic powder
  Freshly ground black pepper to taste (optional)
- 1 can (15 ounces) chickpeas, rinsed
- 1 can (15 ounces) white beans, rinsed
- 1 cup chopped red, yellow, or orange bell pepper
- ½ cup chopped fresh tomatoes
- 1–1½ cups quartered or roughly chopped artichoke hearts (frozen or canned, not marinated in oil)
- ¼ cup chopped or sliced dry-pack sun-dried tomatoes
- ¼ cup sliced green portion of green onion or chives
- ⅓ cup sliced kalamata olives
- ¼ cup chopped fresh basil leaves
- 3 tablespoons raisins or ¼ cup sliced grapes (optional)

In a large bowl, combine the lemon juice, vinegar, syrup, mustard, salt, oregano, garlic powder, and black pepper (if using). Whisk to thoroughly combine. Add the chickpeas, beans, bell pepper, fresh tomatoes, artichoke hearts, sun-dried tomatoes, green onion or chives, olives, basil, and raisins or grapes (if using). Mix well to fully coat with the dressing. Taste, and season with extra salt and black pepper, if desired. Serve, or refrigerate for up to 4 days.

NUTRITIONAL FACTS

Per serving: 275 calories, 15 g protein, 49 g carbohydrates, 10 g sugar, 4 g total fat, 12% calories from fat, 15 g fiber, 801 mg sodium

POPEYE GREEN SALAD

MAKES 4 SERVINGS

Be strong to the finish with this delicious salad! Feel free to substitute other vegetables, such as sliced cucumbers or grated carrots, for the bell pepper or tomatoes or other nuts and seeds in place of the walnuts or pumpkin seeds.

6 cups baby spinach leaves

1 cup sliced red, yellow, or orange bell pepper

½ cup sliced cherry or grape tomatoes

2 tablespoons chopped walnuts or toasted pumpkin seeds

2 tablespoons sliced green onions or chives

½ cup Mango-Hemp Dressing (page 86)

Freshly ground black pepper to taste (optional)

In a large bowl, add the spinach. Distribute the bell pepper, tomatoes, walnuts or seeds, and onions or chives over the spinach. Just before serving, drizzle on the dressing. Add black pepper (if using) to taste, and serve.

NUTRITIONAL FACTS

Per serving (with Mango-Hemp Dressing): 77 calories, 3 g protein, 10 g carbohydrates, 6 g sugar, 4 g total fat, 40% calories from fat, 3 g fiber, 193 mg sodium

OLIVE OYL DINNER SALAD

MAKES 4 SERVINGS

Popeye's met his match with Olive Oyl's salad full of greens, crunchy veggies, and an irresistible dressing!

6 cups mixed greens (boxed mixed greens, a mix of romaine and red leaf lettuce, etc.)

½ cup diced cucumbers

½ cup sliced grapes

½ cup grated carrots

3 tablespoons sliced kalamata olives (can substitute chopped sun-dried tomato)

1–2 tablespoons sliced green onions

½ cup Green Goddess Dressing (page 85)

Sweet Potato Crisps (page 187; optional)

Freshly ground black pepper to taste (optional)

In a large bowl, add the greens. Distribute the cucumbers, grapes, carrots, olives, and onions over the greens. Just before serving, drizzle on the dressing and sprinkle on the Sweet Potato Crisps (if using). Add pepper to taste, if using, and serve.

NUTRITIONAL FACTS

Per serving: 86 calories, 3 g protein, 14 g carbohydrates, 6 g sugar, 3 g total fat, 25% calories from fat, 4 g fiber, 318 mg sodium

GRILLED HUMMUS SANDWICH

MAKES 1 SERVING

Move over, cheese, there's a new grilled sandwich! If you've made your hummus in advance, these sandwiches cook up in just minutes.

⅓ cup Essential Hummus (page 62)

2 slices sprouted grain bread

¼ cup chopped or sliced red bell pepper or ⅓ cup chopped baby spinach

1 tablespoon sliced olives or chopped sun-dried tomatoes

Place a nonstick skillet over medium-high heat. Spread about half of the hummus on one slice of bread, then top with the pepper or spinach and olives or tomatoes. Spread the remaining hummus on the other slice of bread. Close up the sandwich, and place it in the skillet. Cook for 3 to 4 minutes, or until lightly browned. Flip and cook for another 3 to 4 minutes, or until lightly browned. Transfer to a cooling rack (so the underside doesn't soften) to cool slightly, then transfer to a plate and cut in half. Serve.

Shown in color insert pages

NUTRITIONAL FACTS
Per serving: 329 calories, 12 g protein, 49 g carbohydrates, 7 g sugar, 10 g total fat, 26% calories from fat, 9 g fiber, 801 mg sodium

GRILLED NUT BUTTER SANDWICH

MAKES 1 SERVING

For a sweet version of a grilled sandwich, just reach for your favorite nut butter. This will become a favorite for breakfasts or lunches!

2–3 teaspoons almond or other nut butter (can substitute sunflower butter, Wowbutter, or tigernut butter)

2 slices sprouted grain bread

½ cup sliced ripe banana or apple

¼ teaspoon cinnamon

⅓ cup unsweetened applesauce

Place a nonstick skillet over medium-high heat. Spread about half of the nut butter on one slice of bread, then top with the banana or apple and cinnamon. Spread the remaining nut butter on the other slice of bread. Close up the sandwich, and place it in the skillet. Cook for 3 to 4 minutes, or until lightly browned. Flip and cook for another 3 to 4 minutes, or until lightly browned. Transfer to a cooling rack (so the underside doesn't soften) to cool slightly, then transfer to a plate and cut in half. Serve with the applesauce for dipping.

NUTRITIONAL FACTS
Per serving: 332 calories, 9 g protein, 60 g carbohydrates, 20 g sugar, 8 g total fat, 21% calories from fat, 7 g fiber, 412 mg sodium

KALE YEAH! SMASHED WHITE BEANS

MAKES 2 SERVINGS

White beans are versatile in sandwich fillings. They are easy to mash and take on seasonings quite well. This is the first of two smashed white bean sandwich fillings, combining kale and olives.

2 cups torn kale (2 to 3 large leaves, torn from stalk)

1 can (15 ounces) white beans, drained and rinsed

1½ tablespoons tahini

¼ cup sliced kalamata olives

½ teaspoon garlic powder

¼ teaspoon sea salt (see Note)

½ tablespoon fresh thyme or 1 tablespoon fresh chives, chopped (optional)

Freshly ground black pepper to taste (optional)

1½–2 tablespoons red wine vinegar

Place a steamer basket in a large pot with 2" of water. Bring to a boil over high heat. Place the kale in the basket and steam for 1 minute. Drain the kale, press out the excess water, and chop finely. In a mixing bowl, use a fork or your hands to mash the beans. Add the kale, tahini, olives, garlic powder, salt, thyme, and pepper (if using), and 1½ tablespoons of the vinegar. Stir well. Taste, add the remaining ½ tablespoon vinegar if you'd like the extra punch, and season with additional salt and pepper to taste.

NOTE • With the olives, you won't need to add too much salt to this mixture. Start with ¼ teaspoon, and then add more to taste, if you like.

SERVING SUGGESTIONS: Serve on toasted pumpernickel, rye, or whole grain bread; tucked inside whole grain pitas with lettuce, sliced cucumbers, and sliced tomatoes; or rolled in lettuce leaves for green wraps!

NUTRITIONAL FACTS
Per serving: 297 calories, 17 g protein, 41 g carbohydrates, 1 g sugar, 8 g total fat, 24% calories from fat, 11 g fiber, 662 mg sodium

SMASHED WHITE BEANS WITH SPINACH AND SUN-DRIED TOMATOES

MAKES 2 SERVINGS

This second variation pairs sun-dried tomatoes with baby spinach and the enticing flavor of smoked paprika.

1 can (15 ounces) white beans, drained and rinsed

1 cup packed fresh baby spinach leaves

1½ tablespoons lemon juice

1 tablespoon tahini

¼ cup chopped sun-dried tomatoes

½ teaspoon garlic powder

½ teaspoon smoked paprika

¼ teaspoon sea salt (see Note)

2 tablespoons chopped fresh basil (optional; omit if you don't have fresh on hand)

1 tablespoon fresh chives or green onions, chopped

Freshly ground black pepper to taste (optional)

In a mixing bowl, use a fork or your hands to mash the beans. Chop the spinach finely. Add the spinach, lemon juice, tahini, tomatoes, garlic powder, paprika, salt, basil (if using), chives or green onions, and pepper (if using). Stir well. Taste, and season with extra salt and pepper to taste.

NOTE • With the sun-dried tomatoes, you won't need to add too much salt to this mixture. Start with ¼ teaspoon, and then add more to taste, if you like.

SERVING SUGGESTIONS: Serve on toasted pumpernickel, rye, or whole grain bread; tucked inside whole grain pitas with lettuce and sliced bell peppers; or rolled in lettuce leaves for green wraps!

Shown in color insert pages

NUTRITIONAL FACTS
Per serving: 273 calories, 17 g protein, 44 g carbohydrates, 4 g sugar, 5 g total fat, 15% calories from fat, 11 g fiber, 685 mg sodium

SOUPS AND STEWS

BLACK BEAN SOUP WITH SWEET POTATOES

MAKES 4 SERVINGS

This irresistible soup has a touch of sweetness from potatoes. Don't let the number of ingredients intimidate you—they build layers of flavor, but this soup is really quick and easy to make.

1 tablespoon balsamic vinegar

1½–1¾ cups chopped onion

1½ cups combination of chopped red and green bell peppers

1 teaspoon sea salt

Freshly ground black pepper to taste

2 teaspoons cumin seeds

2 teaspoons dried oregano leaves

Rounded ¼ teaspoon allspice

¼ teaspoon red-pepper flakes, or to taste

1–4 tablespoons + 3 cups water

4 medium-large cloves garlic, minced or grated

2 tablespoons tomato paste

2 tablespoons freshly squeezed lime juice

½–1 teaspoon pure maple syrup

4½ cups (about 3 cans, 15 ounces each) black beans, drained and rinsed

1 bay leaf

1½ cups ½" cubes yellow sweet potato (can substitute white potato)

Chopped cilantro (optional)

Extra lime wedges (optional)

In a large pot over medium-high heat, combine the vinegar, onion, bell peppers, salt, black pepper, cumin seeds, oregano, allspice, and red-pepper flakes. Cook for 5 to 7 minutes, or until the onions and red peppers start to soften. Add 1 to 2 tablespoons of water if needed to keep the vegetables from sticking. Add the garlic and stir. Cover, reduce the heat to medium, and cook for another few minutes, until the garlic is softened. If anything is sticking or burning, add another 1 to 2 tablespoons of water. When the garlic is soft, add the tomato paste, lime juice, ½ teaspoon of the syrup, 3½ cups of the beans, and the remaining 3 cups water. Use an immersion blender to puree the soup until it's fairly smooth. Add the bay leaf and sweet potato, increase the heat to high to bring to a boil, then reduce the heat to low and simmer for 20 to 30 minutes. Add the remaining 1 cup black beans. Taste, and add the remaining ½ teaspoon syrup, if desired. Stir, simmer for another few minutes, then serve, seasoning to taste and topping with the cilantro (if using) and lime wedges (if using).

NUTRITIONAL FACTS

Per serving: 368 calories, 19 g protein, 73 g carbohydrates, 10 g sugar, 2 g total fat, 4% calories from fat, 24 g fiber, 1,049 mg sodium

SWEET POTATO BISQUE WITH WHITE BEANS

MAKES 4 SERVINGS

This soup is easy to prepare and the flavors are deep and layered, thanks to the trick of sautéing with balsamic vinegar.

1½ tablespoons balsamic vinegar

2 cups chopped onions

1 cup chopped red pepper (roasted or raw)

1¼ teaspoons sea salt + more to taste

1 teaspoon dried rosemary or 2 teaspoons fresh, roughly chopped

1 teaspoon paprika (can substitute smoked paprika, for extra flavor)

Freshly ground black pepper to taste

3–3½ cups peeled, cubed yellow sweet potatoes

1½–2 teaspoons Dijon mustard

4 cups water

2 cans (15 ounces each) white beans, drained and rinsed

In a soup pot over medium-high heat, combine the vinegar, onions, red pepper, salt, rosemary, paprika, and black pepper. Cover, reduce the heat to medium or medium-low, and cook for 8 to 9 minutes, or until the onions are softened and starting to caramelize. Add the sweet potatoes and mustard, and stir with 1 to 2 tablespoons of the water. Cover and cook for a few minutes. Add the remaining water and increase the heat to high to bring to a boil. Reduce the heat to low, cover, and simmer for 15 to 20 minutes, or until the sweet potatoes are cooked through. Turn off the heat and add 1 cup of the white beans. Use an immersion blender to puree until the bisque is smooth and silky. Add the remaining beans, cover, and simmer for 5 to 10 minutes. Serve.

NUTRITIONAL FACTS

Per serving: 327 calories, 17 g protein, 65 g carbohydrates, 12 g sugar, 1 g total fat, 3% calories from fat, 13 g fiber, 1,044 mg sodium

THAI CORN AND SWEET POTATO STEW

MAKES 4 SERVINGS

This stew is easy to make and is lightly spicy. Try pairing it with brown rice and Soft-Baked Tamari Tofu (page 175).

1   small can (5.5 ounces) light coconut milk

1   cup chopped onion

½   cup chopped celery

2   cups cubed sweet potato (can use frozen)

¾–1 teaspoon sea salt

2   cups water

1½ tablespoons Thai yellow or red curry paste

1½ cups frozen corn kernels

1½ cups chopped red bell pepper

1   package (12–14 ounces) tofu, cut into cubes, or 1 can (14 ounces) black beans, rinsed and drained

2½ tablespoons freshly squeezed lime juice

4–5 cups baby spinach leaves

⅓–½ cup fresh cilantro or Thai basil, chopped

Lime wedges (optional)

In a soup pot over high heat, warm 2 tablespoons of the coconut milk. Add the onion, celery, sweet potato, and ¾ teaspoon of the salt, and sauté for 4 to 5 minutes. Add the water, Thai paste, and remaining coconut milk. Increase the heat to high to bring to a boil. Cover and reduce the heat to medium-low, and let the mixture simmer for 8 to 10 minutes, or until the sweet potato has softened. Turn off the heat, and use an immersion blender to puree the soup base. Add the corn, bell pepper, and tofu or beans, and turn the heat to medium-low. Cover and cook for 3 to 4 minutes to heat through. Add the lime juice, spinach, and cilantro or basil, and stir until the spinach has just wilted. Taste, and season with the remaining ¼ teaspoon salt, if desired. Serve with the lime wedges (if using).

Shown in color insert pages

NUTRITIONAL FACTS
Per serving: 223 calories, 10 g protein, 36 g carbohydrates, 11 g sugar, 7 g total fat, 26% calories from fat, 6 g fiber, 723 mg sodium

ROBUST CRIMSON BEAN STEW

MAKES 4 SERVINGS

This is one of those soups that you'll return to time and time again. It's easy, really nourishing, and delicious any time of year.

1   cup chopped red onion

2   teaspoons dried oregano

1   teaspoon dried rosemary

1   teaspoon Dijon mustard
    Freshly ground black pepper to taste

2   tablespoons + 2½ cups water

2   cups cubed yellow or red potatoes

½   cup dry black beluga or French lentils (can substitute green or brown lentils)

½   cup uncooked brown or red rice (can substitute quinoa)

3   cloves minced or grated garlic

1   can (28 ounces) crushed tomatoes (see Tomatoes Note)

1   can (15 ounces) adzuki, black, or kidney beans, rinsed and drained

1–1½   cups chopped red peppers (see Red Pepper Note)

2   tablespoons vegan Worcestershire sauce

¼   teaspoon sea salt

In an instant pot set on the sauté function, combine the onion, oregano, rosemary, mustard, black pepper, and 2 tablespoons of the water. Cook for 3 to 4 minutes. Turn off the sauté function and stir in the potatoes, lentils, rice, garlic, tomatoes, beans, and remaining 2½ cups water. Cook on high pressure for 15 minutes, and either release the pressure manually or let it naturally release. Add the red peppers, Worcestershire sauce, and salt to the instant pot. Stir, replace the cover, and let sit for 5 to 8 minutes. Taste, season as desired, and serve.

STOVETOP VARIATION: In a large pot over medium-high heat, combine the onion, oregano, rosemary, mustard, black pepper, and 2 tablespoons of the water. Cook for 4 to 5 minutes, then add the potatoes, lentils, rice, garlic, tomatoes, beans, and remaining 2½ cups water. Increase the heat to high, bring to a boil, and reduce the heat to low. Cook for 30 to 35 minutes, or until the rice is fully cooked through. Add the red peppers, Worcestershire sauce, and salt. Stir, and cook for another 5 minutes. Once the peppers are just tender, taste, season as desired, and serve.

TOMATOES NOTE • If you prefer a smoother consistency or you only have whole or diced tomatoes on hand, use an immersion blender to puree the tomatoes right in the can. Just pour off a couple inches of the juice (and reserve for the recipe), then immerse the blender and puree until smooth.

RED PEPPER NOTE • Adding the red peppers later in the cooking process lets them retain more texture. You can add them earlier in the cooking process, with the tomatoes and beans, if you like.

NUTRITIONAL FACTS
Per serving: 596 calories, 29 g protein, 120 g carbohydrates, 11 g sugar, 2 g total fat, 3% calories from fat, 28 g fiber, 523 mg sodium

SPUD-LOVERS' LENTIL CHILI

MAKES 6 SERVINGS

Chock-full of hearty lentils, along with two types of potatoes, this is a meal in a bowl.

1½ cups onions, finely chopped

2 cups cubed red or yellow potatoes (not russet)

2 cups cubed sweet potatoes (can use frozen)

3–4 large cloves garlic, minced

1¼ teaspoons sea salt

1 tablespoon chili powder

1 teaspoon dried oregano

1 teaspoon paprika or smoked paprika

1 teaspoon ground cumin

½ teaspoon cinnamon

2 tablespoons finely chopped pitted dates

2–5 tablespoons + 3½ cups water

1 cup dried red lentils

1 cup dried green lentils

1 can (28 ounces) crushed tomatoes

2–3 tablespoons freshly squeezed lime juice

Lime wedges

In a large pot over medium heat, combine the onions, potatoes, sweet potatoes, garlic, salt, chili powder, oregano, paprika, cumin, cinnamon, dates, and 2 to 3 tablespoons of the water, and stir. Cover and cook for 6 to 8 minutes, stirring occasionally. Reduce the heat if the mixture is sticking to the bottom of the pot, and add 1 to 2 tablespoons of water. Rinse the red and green lentils. Add the lentils, tomatoes, and remaining 3½ cups water to the pot, and stir to combine. Increase the heat to bring to a boil. Reduce the heat to low, cover, and simmer for 40 minutes or longer, until the green lentils are fully cooked through and softened. Stir in the lime juice (adjusting to taste), and serve portions with lime wedges.

NUTRITIONAL FACTS

Per serving: 337 calories, 19 g protein, 66 g carbohydrates, 11 g sugar, 2 g total fat, 4% calories from fat, 17 g fiber, 698 mg sodium

ROASTED TOMATO AND SWEET POTATO SOUP

MAKES 4 SERVINGS

Let the oven do the work of creating the base for this soup—then blend and you're ready to dig in!

1½ cups peeled, quartered onion (roughly 1 large onion)

4 cups cubed sweet potato (roughly 1–1¼ pounds before peeling)

4 cups (about 1½ pounds) quartered Roma or other tomatoes, juices squeezed out

1½ teaspoons dried basil

1½ teaspoons dried oregano

1 tablespoon balsamic vinegar

1 teaspoon blackstrap molasses

Freshly ground black pepper to taste

1⅛ teaspoons sea salt

2¼–2½ cups water

¼ cup chopped fresh basil (optional)

Preheat the oven to 450°F.

In a large baking dish, combine the onion, sweet potato, tomatoes, basil, oregano, vinegar, molasses, pepper, and 1 teaspoon of the salt. Cook for 40 to 50 minutes, stirring a couple of times, until the sweet potatoes are softened and the mixture is becoming caramelized. Transfer the vegetables and any juices they've released in the pan to a medium soup pot, add 2¼ cups of the water and the remaining ⅛ teaspoon salt, and use an immersion blender to puree. (Alternatively, you can transfer everything to a blender to puree.) Blend to the desired smoothness, using the additional ¼ cup water if needed. Stir in fresh basil, if using, and serve.

SERVING IDEA: Try adding ½ to 1 cup of cooked brown rice and pureeing for a thicker, heartier soup.

IDEA: Leftovers of this soup make a fantastic pasta sauce!

NUTRITIONAL FACTS
Per serving: 152 calories, 4 g protein, 35 g carbohydrates, 14 g sugar, 0.4 g total fat, 2% calories from fat, 5 g fiber, 648 mg sodium

GREEK LENTIL AND WHITE BEAN SOUP WITH OLIVE AND TOMATO GREMOLATA

MAKES 5 SERVINGS

This soup combines the heartiness of beans and lentils with subtle spices.

Gremolata Garnish (see Gremolata Note)

- 1 teaspoon lemon zest
- 2–3 tablespoons finely chopped fresh parsley or 1–2 tablespoons finely chopped fresh mint
- 2 tablespoons finely chopped kalamata or dry cured olives
- 3–4 tablespoons finely chopped tomatoes

Soup

- 1½ cups chopped onion
- ½ cup diced celery
- 4 teaspoons dried oregano
- ½ teaspoon allspice
- ⅛ teaspoon ground cinnamon
- 1¼ teaspoons sea salt
  Freshly ground black pepper
- 3 tablespoons + 4 cups water
- 1 cup dried red lentils
- 3 cups cooked white beans
- 1 medium or large clove garlic (see Garlic Note)
- ¼ cup freshly squeezed lemon juice
- ½–1 teaspoon lemon zest

To prepare the gremolata: In a small bowl, combine the lemon zest, parsley or mint, olives, and tomatoes. Stir thoroughly and set aside.

To prepare the soup: In a soup pot over medium-high heat, combine the onion, celery, oregano, allspice, cinnamon, salt, pepper, and 3 tablespoons of the water. Stir, cover, and cook for 5 to 6 minutes, stirring once. Add the lentils, 2 cups of the white beans, and the remaining 4 cups water. Increase the heat to bring the mixture to a boil. Reduce the heat to low, cover, and simmer for 20 minutes.

Turn off the heat and use an immersion blender to puree until smooth. Stir in the remaining 1 cup white beans and use a kitchen rasp to grate the garlic into the soup. Add the lemon juice and zest, and stir. Taste, and add additional salt or pepper if desired. Top each portion with a few teaspoons of the gremolata and serve.

GREMOLATA NOTE • If you don't want to use the gremolata, try topping with a sprinkle of nutritional yeast.

GARLIC NOTE • If you prefer to cook the garlic, simply add it along with the onion and celery, taking care not to let it scorch. You can use 2 cloves if you're adding it earlier, as the flavor will mellow with cooking.

Shown in color insert pages

NUTRITIONAL FACTS
Per serving: 304 calories, 21 g protein, 55 g carbohydrates, 4 g sugar, 1 g total fat, 4% calories from fat, 14 g fiber, 957 mg sodium

JAMAICAN STEW

MAKES 4 SERVINGS

This hearty stew combines earthy spices with a gingery kick and a pop of lime. The combination is delicious!

1½ cups chopped onions

3–4 cups cubed plantains (see Note; can substitute sweet potatoes)

1¼ teaspoons sea salt

1½ teaspoons ground coriander

½ teaspoon ground cumin

½ teaspoon ground turmeric

1 teaspoon dried thyme

½ teaspoon ground allspice

¼ teaspoon crushed red-pepper flakes (or to taste)

1 small can (5.5 ounces) light coconut milk

3½ cups water

2 cans (15 ounces each) black beans or adzuki beans, rinsed and drained

3 cups cauliflower florets

2 tablespoons freshly grated ginger

3 tablespoons freshly squeezed lime juice

3 cups baby spinach leaves

¼ cup freshly chopped cilantro (optional)

Lime wedges for serving

In a large pot over medium or medium-high heat, combine the onion, plantains, salt, coriander, cumin, turmeric, thyme, allspice, red-pepper flakes, and a few tablespoons of the coconut milk. Cook for 6 to 7 minutes, stirring occasionally. Add the water, beans, cauliflower, ginger, and remaining coconut milk. Increase the heat to high to bring to a boil, then reduce the heat to low, cover, and cook for 12 to 15 minutes, or until the plantains are cooked through. Add the lime juice, spinach, and cilantro (if using), and stir just until the spinach wilts. Serve immediately, with the lime wedges.

NOTE • When plantains are less ripe (more greenish), they are less sweet and taste somewhat like a potato crossed with a yellow sweet potato. For this recipe, use plantains that aren't green, but that aren't fully ripe, with too much brown, either. Also, while they look like bananas, plantains cannot be peeled like bananas. Instead, trim the ends and then use your hands or a knife to loosen and pry back the peels.

Shown in color insert pages

NUTRITIONAL FACTS
Per serving: 426 calories, 16 g protein, 88 g carbohydrates, 22 g sugar, 5 g total fat, 9% calories from fat, 22 g fiber, 1,053 mg sodium

CAULIFLOWER CHILI

MAKES 5 SERVINGS

Minced carrot and cauliflower add great texture to this dish, and the flavor is wonderful.

2   cups thickly sliced carrot

½   large or 1 full small head cauliflower

4   or 5 cloves garlic, minced

1   tablespoon balsamic vinegar

1½ cups diced onion

1   teaspoon sea salt

1½ tablespoons mild chili powder

1   tablespoon cocoa powder

2   teaspoons ground cumin

2   teaspoons dried oregano

⅛   teaspoon allspice

¼   teaspoon crushed red-pepper flakes (or to taste)

1   can (28 ounces) crushed tomatoes

1   can (15 ounces) pinto beans, rinsed and drained

1   can (15 ounces) kidney beans or black beans, rinsed and drained

½   cup water

    Lime wedges

In a food processor, combine the carrot, cauliflower, and garlic, and pulse until finely minced. (Alternatively, you could mince by hand.) In a large pot over medium heat, combine the vinegar, onion, salt, chili powder, cocoa, cumin, oregano, allspice, and red-pepper flakes. Cook for 3 to 4 minutes, stirring occasionally. Add the minced carrot, cauliflower, and garlic, and cook for 5 to 6 minutes, stirring occasionally. Add the tomatoes, pinto and kidney beans, and water, and stir to combine. Increase the heat to high to bring to a boil. Reduce the heat to low, cover, and simmer for 25 minutes. Taste, and season as desired. Serve with lime wedges.

NUTRITIONAL FACTS

Per serving: 237 calories, 13 g protein, 45 g carbohydrates, 13 g sugar, 3 g total fat, 10% calories from fat, 15 g fiber, 1,036 mg sodium

GOLDEN LENTIL-PEA SOUP

MAKES 6 SERVINGS

With the lightness of red lentils and sweet potatoes, this is unlike any pea soup you've tasted. Don't skip the apple cider vinegar finish at the end—it works!

1 cup diced onion

1 cup chopped celery

1 tablespoon smoked paprika

1 teaspoon dried rosemary

1 teaspoon ground cumin

¼ teaspoon allspice

¼ teaspoon sea salt

2–3 tablespoons + 4 cups water

4 cups chopped yellow sweet potato (or 2 cups chopped sweet potato and 2 cups chopped carrot)

1½ cups dried red lentils

1 cup dried yellow split peas

2 cups vegetable broth

1½ tablespoons apple cider vinegar

In a large soup pot over medium-high heat, combine the onion, celery, paprika, rosemary, cumin, allspice, salt, and 2 to 3 tablespoons of the water, and stir. Cook for 8 to 9 minutes, then add the potato, lentils, split peas, broth, and the remaining 4 cups of water. Stir to combine. Increase the heat to high to bring to a boil. Reduce the heat to low, cover, and simmer for 40 to 45 minutes, or until the peas are completely softened. Stir in the apple cider vinegar, season with additional salt and pepper if desired, and serve.

NUTRITIONAL FACTS
Per serving: 340 calories, 21 g protein, 64 g carbohydrates, 8 g sugar, 1 g total fat, 3% calories from fat, 20 g fiber, 363 mg sodium

LENTIL MINESTRONE

MAKES 5 SERVINGS

This delicious minestrone is a perfect meal, complete with veggies, beans, and whole grain pasta.

3 tablespoons white wine or 1–2 tablespoons water

1 cup diced onion

1 cup diced carrots

½ cup diced zucchini (can substitute celery)

3 large cloves garlic, minced

2 teaspoons dried oregano

1 teaspoon dried basil

½ teaspoon fennel seeds

1 teaspoon sea salt

1 jar (24 ounces) strained tomatoes (can substitute one 28-ounce can crushed tomatoes)

½ cup dried green lentils

1 can (15 ounces) kidney beans, rinsed and drained

3 cups water

1 fresh or dried bay leaf

1 cup dry cut pasta (such as penne, rotini, or macaroni)

1 cup fresh or frozen green beans

½–1 teaspoon pure maple syrup (optional)

In a large pot over medium-high heat, combine the wine or water, onion, carrots, zucchini, garlic, oregano, basil, fennel, and salt. Stir and cook for 4 to 5 minutes, reducing the heat if the veggies are sticking or burning. Add the tomatoes, lentils, beans, water, and bay leaf. Bring to a boil, then reduce the heat to low, cover, and cook for 30 minutes. Add the pasta, and cook for 5 minutes. Add the green beans, and cook for another 3 to 5 minutes, until the pasta is tender and the green beans are just cooked through. Taste, and add the syrup to taste (if using). Serve.

NUTRITIONAL FACTS
Per serving: 386 calories, 20 g protein, 72 g carbohydrates, 11 g sugar, 3 g total fat, 6% calories from fat, 15 g fiber, 960 mg sodium

CAULI-CURRY BEAN SOUP

MAKES 8 SERVINGS

This soup is easy and delicious. Save some for later; the flavors just get better!

2 cups chopped onion	⅛ teaspoon ground cinnamon
1½ cups chopped carrot or sweet potato	4–5 tablespoons + 4 cups water
1½ tablespoons curry powder (or to taste; use more if you really love curry)	3–4 cups cauliflower florets
	1 can (15 ounces) chickpeas, rinsed and drained
1¼ teaspoons sea salt	1 can (15 ounces) adzuki or black beans, rinsed and drained
Freshly ground black pepper to taste	1 cup dried red lentils
1 teaspoon mustard seeds	1 can (28 ounces) crushed tomatoes (see Note)
1 teaspoon ground cumin	1 tablespoon grated fresh ginger
1 teaspoon ground turmeric	1–2 teaspoons pure maple syrup (optional)
¼ teaspoon ground cardamom	

In a large pot over medium-high heat, combine the onion, carrot or sweet potato, curry powder, salt, pepper, mustard seeds, cumin, turmeric, cardamom, cinnamon, and 3 tablespoons of the water. Stir, cover, and cook for 4 to 5 minutes, stirring occasionally. (Add another 1 to 2 tablespoons of water if needed to keep the vegetables and spices from sticking.) Add the cauliflower, chickpeas, beans, lentils, tomatoes, and remaining 4 cups water. Stir and increase the heat to high to bring to a boil. Reduce the heat to low, cover, and simmer for 15 to 20 minutes. Stir in the ginger and syrup (if using). Season to taste, and serve.

NOTE • If you only have whole or diced tomatoes, you can puree them in a blender or right in the can using an immersion blender. Just pour off a couple inches of the juice (and reserve for the recipe), then immerse the blender and puree until smooth.

NUTRITIONAL FACTS
Per serving: 226 calories, 14 g protein, 42 g carbohydrates, 7 g sugar, 2 g total fat, 8% calories from fat, 13 g fiber, 577 mg sodium

HODGEPODGE STEW

MAKES 4 SERVINGS

This stew combines simple ingredients to make an easy and nutritious meal.

3 tablespoons water

2 cups roughly chopped onion

2–2½ cups cauliflower florets (see Cauliflower Note)

1½ cups thickly sliced carrots

1 teaspoon dried thyme leaves

1 teaspoon dried savory or rosemary leaves (or ½ teaspoon each)

1 teaspoon mustard seeds

½ teaspoon dill seed (optional)

¼ teaspoon sea salt

3 tablespoons spelt or other flour

2 cups vegetable stock

3 cups cubed potatoes (can substitute sweet potatoes)

1 can (15 ounces) kidney beans, drained and rinsed (see Kidney Beans Note)

1½ cups low-fat nondairy milk

1 cup chopped green beans or frozen green peas

2 tablespoons nutritional yeast (optional)

In a large pot over medium-high heat, combine the water, onion, cauliflower, carrots, thyme, savory or rosemary, mustard seeds, dill (if using), and salt. Cook for 3 to 4 minutes, stirring a few times. Add the flour and stir frequently for another few minutes, to help cook out the raw flavor of the flour. Add a splash of the vegetable stock if needed to prevent sticking. Add the remainder of the stock gradually, starting with ¼ to ½ cup and stirring it into the flour steadily, allowing the flour and stock to thicken together. Let the mixture bubble, and then continue adding the stock. Add the potatoes and beans, and let the mixture come to a boil. Reduce the heat to medium-low, cover the pot, and cook for 15 minutes, or until the potatoes are tender when pierced. Add the milk, green beans or peas, and yeast (if using). Heat through for 4 to 5 minutes, then serve.

CAULIFLOWER NOTE • Don't have any cauliflower on hand? Try substituting a combination of thickly sliced celery and parsnip or turnip.

KIDNEY BEANS NOTE • Kidney beans add a lovely color, but you can substitute chickpeas, cannellini beans, or black beans.

NUTRITIONAL FACTS
Per serving: 250 calories, 10 g protein, 51 g carbohydrates, 11 g sugar, 2 g total fat, 6% calories from fat, 9 g fiber, 558 mg sodium

MAINS

MARINARA SAUCE

MAKES 5 SERVINGS (5 TO 5½ CUPS)

Making your own marinara sauce is surprisingly easy, especially if you use an instant pot or other pressure cooker.

2 tablespoons red or white wine

3 cups chopped onion

½–¾ cup diced carrot

1 teaspoon sea salt

Few pinches freshly ground black pepper (or more to taste)

6–7 cloves garlic, minced

3 pounds chopped ripe tomatoes (8–9 cups)

2–3 sliced, pitted dates (about 1½ tablespoons)

½ cup loosely packed fresh basil (can substitute 2 tablespoons fresh chopped oregano)

In a large pot over high heat, combine the wine, onion, carrot, salt, and pepper. Stir and let cook for 4 to 5 minutes, then add the garlic, tomatoes, dates, and basil. Bring the mixture to a boil, stirring frequently. Once it has reached a boil, reduce the heat to low or medium-low, cover, and let simmer for 40 minutes. Use an immersion blender to puree the sauce to the desired consistency. Taste, and add extra salt or pepper to taste. Serve with the pasta of your choice. (Try it in the Marinara Pasta with Artichokes and Olives.)

INSTANT POT VARIATION: In an instant pot set to the sauté function, combine the wine, onion, carrot, salt, and pepper. Let cook for 3 to 4 minutes, stirring occasionally. Turn off the sauté function, then add the garlic, tomatoes, dates, and basil. Set the instant pot to high pressure for 20 minutes. Manually release the pressure, or let it release naturally. Use an immersion blender to puree the sauce to the desired consistency. Taste, and add extra salt or pepper to taste. Serve with pasta of your choice. (Try in Marinara Pasta with Artichokes and Olives.)

NUTRITIONAL FACTS
Per serving: 98 calories, 4 g protein, 21 g carbohydrates, 11 g sugar, 0.5 g total fat, 4% calories from fat, 3 g fiber, 505 mg sodium

MARINARA PASTA WITH ARTICHOKES AND OLIVES

MAKES 5 SERVINGS

If you've already prepared our Marinara Sauce, this meal comes together in minutes!

1½ pounds dry pasta	½ cup sliced kalamata olives
1 batch Marinara Sauce (see Note)	¼ teaspoon sea salt (adjust to taste)
2–3 cups chopped artichoke hearts (frozen or canned, not marinated in oil)	Few pinches freshly ground black pepper (adjust to taste)
	⅓ cup julienned fresh basil leaves

Cook the pasta according to package directions. Once the pasta is cooked, drain but don't rinse it. Return the pasta to the pot and place it over low heat. Add the Marinara Sauce, artichoke hearts, olives, and salt and pepper to taste. Stir gently to heat through. Once everything is well heated, add the basil just to wilt, and serve. Season with additional salt and pepper to taste.

NOTE • If you like a "saucy" pasta, you'll probably want to use the full batch of sauce. But you can always start with less and add more as you go.

IDEA: Instead of olives, try chopped sun-dried tomatoes. Instead of (or in addition to) artichoke hearts, try chopped roasted bell peppers or roasted cauliflower.

NUTRITIONAL FACTS
Per serving (including full batch of Marinara Sauce): 741 calories, 27 g protein, 146 g carbohydrates, 14 g sugar, 6 g total fat, 6% calories from fat, 16 g fiber, 911 mg sodium

RIGHTEOUS LASAGNA

MAKES 6 SERVINGS

For real, this is one righteous lasagna. No cheese needed. It is straight-up delicious!

1 pound portobello (5 or 6 medium-large), brown, or white mushrooms

1 tablespoon balsamic vinegar

½ tablespoon tamari

1 teaspoon Dijon mustard

¼ teaspoon smoked paprika

Few pinches lemon pepper or freshly ground black pepper (or more to taste)

5 cups (about 1½ jars) good quality, low-sodium pasta sauce

1 package (12 ounces) ready-bake lasagna noodles (see Note)

1 batch Warm Cheesy Sweet Potato Dip (page 66)

1 tablespoon chopped fresh thyme

Preheat the oven to broil. Line a baking sheet with parchment paper.

Clean the mushrooms with a damp paper towel, and if using portobellos, scrape the gills from the undersides and discard. Slice the mushrooms. In a large bowl, whisk together the balsamic, tamari, mustard, paprika, and pepper. Add the mushrooms and toss to coat. Transfer the mushrooms to the prepared baking sheet. Broil for 7 to 9 minutes, or until the mushrooms reduce a little and get some color. Remove and let cool while preparing the lasagna.

Preheat the oven to 375°F. Spread 1 cup of the pasta sauce over the bottom of a 9" x 13" lasagna dish. Cover the sauce with 3 or 4 noodles along the length of the dish. Spread roughly half of the sweet potato dip over the noodles. Top with 4 or 5 more noodles placed in the opposite direction in the pan. (You may need to break the noodles to fit.) Layer on about 1½ cups of sauce and the mushrooms. Sprinkle the thyme over the mushrooms. Top with another 4 or 5 noodles along the length of the dish and the remainder of the pasta sauce, followed by the remainder of the sweet potato dip. Cover the dish tightly with foil. Bake for 50 to 55 minutes, or until the noodles are fully cooked when pierced. Remove from the oven and let rest for 10 minutes before slicing and serving.

NOTE • Using ready-bake noodles makes lasagna prep a lot easier. However, you do need to use a little extra sauce to soften the noodles. If you're using standard lasagna noodles, parboil them until they're just al dente before draining and using them in the lasagna.

NUTRITIONAL FACTS
Per serving: 459 calories, 16 g protein, 80 g carbohydrates, 18 g sugar, 8 g total fat, 16% calories from fat, 10 g fiber, 463 mg sodium

MIGHTY MUSHROOM BURGERS

MAKES 4 SERVINGS

Portobello mushrooms make excellent veggie burgers. They have a meaty texture, absorb seasonings well, and are quick and easy to prepare.

2 tablespoons balsamic vinegar

1 tablespoon natural ketchup

1 tablespoon vegan Worcestershire sauce

1 teaspoon Dijon mustard

½ teaspoon garlic powder

½ teaspoon dried oregano

8 medium-large portobello mushrooms

Pinch of sea salt (optional)

Pinch of freshly ground black pepper (optional)

Serving Ideas (optional):

Whole grain hamburger buns

Condiments of choice (ketchup, mustard, BBQ sauce)

Spreads: Green-with-Envy Guacamole (page 67) or Avocado Hummus (page 68)

In a large bowl, whisk together the vinegar, ketchup, Worcestershire sauce, mustard, garlic powder, and oregano. Remove the stems from the mushrooms, and gently wipe the mushroom caps clean with a damp paper towel. Using a spoon, scrape the gills from the undersides of the mushrooms, discarding the scrapings. Add the mushroom caps to the marinade and gently turn to coat evenly. If you have time, let the mushrooms marinate for 30 minutes or more.

Preheat the grill to high or medium-high heat (see Note). Place the mushrooms on the grill and sprinkle on a pinch of salt and pepper (if using). Grill for 5 to 7 minutes on the first side, until grill marks have formed. Turn the mushroom caps and cook for another 3 to 4 minutes, until cooked through. Serve on burger buns with fixings.

NOTE • If you don't have a grill, you can bake the mushrooms on a baking sheet lined with parchment paper. Preheat the oven to 450°F, and bake for 12 to 15 minutes, turning once. The mushrooms will release their juices as they cook; turn the mushroom caps once or twice to coat in those juices. To brown the mushrooms, set the oven to broil for a couple of minutes. The mushrooms will reduce and caramelize even more.

Shown in color insert pages

NUTRITIONAL FACTS
Per serving (2 mushroom caps, without buns or toppings): 49 calories, 4 g protein, 9 g carbohydrates, 5 g sugar, 1 g total fat, 12% calories from fat, 3 g fiber, 120 mg sodium

LOADED SWEET POTATOES

MAKES 4 SERVINGS

Try this version, and then next time switch it up with your own favorite bean and vegetable combination.

3 pounds sweet potatoes (can substitute white potatoes)

1 can (15 ounces) black beans, drained and rinsed (can substitute another bean)

3 cups cauliflower florets or broccoli, steamed (or frozen, thawed)

¼ cup diced red or yellow bell pepper

¼ cup thinly sliced green onions

Few pinches of sea salt

Few pinches of freshly ground black pepper

1 batch Green-with-Envy Guacamole (page 67)

Preheat the oven to 450°F. Line a baking sheet with parchment paper.

Wash the potatoes and place them, whole, unpeeled, and unpierced, on the prepared baking sheet. Bake for 45 to 60 minutes, or until tender. Remove and let cool. When the potatoes are cool enough to handle, slice them in half. (If you baked them in advance and they have been refrigerated, place in the oven at 400°F for about 10 minutes to reheat.) Top the warm potato halves with the beans, cauliflower or broccoli, bell pepper, onions, salt, and black pepper. Return to the oven for another 5 minutes to heat the toppings. Top each potato with guacamole, and serve.

OPTION: For a spicy version, combine the beans with ½ to ¾ cup of salsa.

NUTRITIONAL FACTS

Per serving: 440 calories, 15 g protein, 77 g carbohydrates, 17 g sugar, 10 g total fat, 20% calories from fat, 22 g fiber, 898 mg sodium

BBQ BEAN BURGERS

MAKES 8 BURGERS

Fire up the grill, it's time for burgers! The extra flavor comes from barbeque sauce, smoked paprika, and vegan Worcestershire sauce. These are a cinch to make!

2 cups sliced carrots

1 medium-large clove garlic, quartered

1 can (15 ounces) kidney beans, rinsed and drained

1 cup cooked, cooled brown rice

¼ cup barbecue sauce

½ tablespoon vegan Worcestershire sauce

½ tablespoon Dijon mustard

Scant ½ teaspoon sea salt

¼–½ teaspoon smoked paprika

1 tablespoon chopped fresh thyme

1¼ cups rolled oats

In a food processor, combine the carrots and garlic. Pulse until minced. Add the beans, rice, barbecue sauce, Worcestershire sauce, mustard, salt, paprika, and thyme. Puree until well combined. Once the mixture is fairly smooth, add the oats and pulse to combine. Chill the mixture for 30 minutes, if possible.

Preheat the oven to 400°F. Line a baking sheet with parchment paper.

Use an ice cream scoop to scoop the mixture onto the prepared baking sheet, flattening to shape it into patties. Bake for about 20 minutes, flipping the burgers halfway through. Alternatively, you can cook the burgers in a nonstick skillet over medium heat for 6 to 8 minutes per side, or until golden brown.

SERVING IDEAS: Serve on whole grain buns, in pitas, or in lettuce wraps.

OPTION: Shape this mixture into balls to serve with spaghetti or to make "meatball sandwiches." Use a small cookie scoop and place the "meatballs" on a parchment-lined baking sheet. (This recipe will make 30 to 35 balls.) Bake at 400°F for 20 to 25 minutes, or until they are firm.

NUTRITIONAL FACTS
Per burger: 152 calories, 6 g protein, 29 g carbohydrates, 6 g sugar, 2 g total fat, 9% calories from fat, 5 g fiber, 347 mg sodium

EASY LENTIL BURGERS

MAKES 5 SERVINGS (10 BURGERS)

Everything goes into the food processor, and you're ready to cook in minutes!

1   medium-large clove garlic

2   tablespoons tamari

2   tablespoons tomato paste

1   tablespoon red wine
    vinegar

1½ tablespoons tahini

2   tablespoons fresh thyme or
    oregano

2   teaspoons onion powder

¼   teaspoon sea salt

    Few pinches freshly ground black
    pepper

3   cups cooked brown lentils

1   cup toasted breadcrumbs
    (see Note)

½   cup rolled oats

In a food processor, combine the garlic, tamari, tomato paste, vinegar, tahini, thyme or oregano, onion powder, salt, pepper, and 1½ cups of the lentils. Puree until fairly smooth. Add the breadcrumbs, rolled oats, and the remaining 1½ cups of lentils. Pulse a few times. At this stage you're looking for a sticky texture that will hold together when pressed. If the mixture is still a little crumbly, pulse a few more times.

Preheat the oven to 400°F. Line a baking sheet with parchment paper.

Use an ice cream scoop to scoop the mixture onto the prepared baking sheet, flattening to shape into patties. Bake for about 20 minutes, flipping the burgers halfway through. Alternatively, you can cook the burgers in a non-stick skillet over medium heat for 4 to 5 minutes per side, or until golden brown.

SERVING IDEAS: Serve on whole grain burger buns with fixings, in whole grain pitas, or on top of a salad.

NOTE • Make your own breadcrumbs at home by processing heels and scraps of bread in a food processor until they have been reduced to small crumbs. Line a baking sheet with parchment paper and spread the crumbs on it evenly. Bake at 375°F for 10 to 15 minutes, or until golden, stirring a couple of times. (Watch them closely while they're toasting, as they can burn quickly.) Once golden, turn off the oven and let the crumbs sit in the residual heat for another 10 minutes (unless they are already browned; if so, remove them from the heat and let them cool on the stovetop). Use them right away, or freeze in an airtight container.

NUTRITIONAL FACTS
Per burger: 148 calories, 8 g protein, 24 g carbohydrates, 1 g sugar, 2 g total fat, 13% calories from fat, 5 g fiber, 369 mg sodium

SUNSHINE BURGERS

MAKES 10 BURGERS

Let the sun shine in with these bright and easy burgers! So easy to make and so tasty, you'll love them.

- 2 cups sliced raw carrots
- 1 large clove garlic, sliced or quartered
- 2 cans (15 ounces each) chickpeas, rinsed and drained
- ¼ cup sliced dry-packed sun-dried tomatoes
- 2 tablespoons tahini

- 1 teaspoon red wine vinegar or apple cider vinegar
- 1 teaspoon smoked paprika
- ½ teaspoon dried rosemary
- ½ teaspoon ground cumin
- ½ teaspoon sea salt
- 1 cup rolled oats

In a food processor, combine the carrots and garlic. Pulse several times to mince. Add the chickpeas, tomatoes, tahini, vinegar, paprika, rosemary, cumin, and salt. Puree until well combined, scraping down the sides of the bowl once or twice. Add the oats, and pulse briefly to combine. Refrigerate the mixture for 30 minutes, if possible.

Preheat the oven to 400°F. Line a baking sheet with parchment paper.

Use an ice cream scoop to scoop the mixture onto the prepared baking sheet, flattening to shape it into patties. Bake for 18 to 20 minutes, flipping the burgers halfway through. Alternatively, you can cook the burgers in a nonstick skillet over medium heat for 6 to 8 minutes per side, or until golden brown. Serve.

SERVING IDEA: Instead of serving on buns, try serving in crispy romaine leaves!

NUTRITIONAL FACTS
Per burger: 137 calories, 6 g protein, 21 g carbohydrates, 4 g sugar, 4 g total fat, 23% calories from fat, 6 g fiber, 278 mg sodium

CREAMY LEMON–TAHINI PASTA WITH SPINACH

MAKES 4 SERVINGS

This sauce takes just minutes to bring together. It's one of the easiest pasta sauces, yet it's so zesty and delicious!

1 pound dry pasta (see Pasta Note)	1–2 medium cloves garlic
⅓ cup freshly squeezed lemon juice	2 teaspoons pure maple syrup
¾ teaspoon sea salt	Few pinches freshly ground black pepper (or more to taste)
1½ teaspoons chickpea miso (or other mild-flavored miso)	2–4 tablespoons water
2 tablespoons tahini	½ teaspoon lemon zest
¼ cup unsweetened applesauce	5 ounces fresh baby spinach (see Spinach Note)

Cook the pasta according to package directions. Meanwhile, prepare the sauce. In a blender, combine the lemon juice, salt, miso, tahini, applesauce, garlic, syrup, pepper, and 2 tablespoons of the water. Puree until smooth, adding the additional 2 tablespoons water if needed. Once the pasta is ready, drain but don't rinse it. Return the pasta to the pot and place it over low heat. Add the sauce, lemon zest, and spinach, and gently heat through. As soon as the spinach is wilted, serve.

PASTA NOTE • This recipe works well with cut pasta, like penne or rotini, or longer noodles, like spaghetti or linguine.

SPINACH NOTE • Feel free to use more than 5 ounces of spinach, if you like. Also, instead of spinach, you can use chopped chard or kale (kale will take longer to wilt), or steamed broccoli or cauliflower.

IDEA: For a heartier pasta, add 1 to 1½ cups of cooked white beans when you add the spinach.

Shown in color insert pages

NUTRITIONAL FACTS
Per serving: 571 calories, 21 g protein, 105 g carbohydrates, 6 g sugar, 7 g total fat, 11% calories from fat, 8 g fiber, 563 mg sodium

MISO RICE PATTIES

MAKES 9 PATTIES

Paired with a great salad and creamy dressing, like Mango-Hemp Dressing (page 86), along with roasted potatoes, tofu, or tempeh, this makes a beautiful meal.

- 2 tablespoons chickpea miso (or other mild-flavored miso)
- ¾ cup sliced green onions (mostly green portion)
- 2 tablespoons ground white chia seeds
- 2 teaspoons red wine vinegar or apple cider vinegar
- 1 medium-large clove garlic, quartered
- Rounded ¼ teaspoon sea salt
- ⅛ teaspoon crushed red-pepper flakes (use more if you like heat)
- 5 cups cooked and cooled brown rice
- ½ cup rolled oats
- ¼ cup + 2 tablespoons almond meal

In a food processor, combine the miso, onions, chia, vinegar, garlic, salt, red-pepper flakes, and 2 cups of the rice. Puree until fairly well incorporated. Add the rolled oats, almond meal, and the remaining 3 cups rice, and pulse to combine. Refrigerate the mixture for 30 minutes or more.

Preheat the oven to 425°F and line a baking sheet with parchment paper.

Use an ice cream scoop to scoop the mixture onto the prepared baking sheet, flattening to shape into patties. Bake for about 20 minutes, flipping the patties halfway through. Alternatively, you can cook the patties in a nonstick skillet over medium heat for 4 to 5 minutes per side, or until golden brown. Serve with Balsamic Drizzle (page 83) or other sauces or condiments of choice.

NUTRITIONAL FACTS
Per patty: 204 calories, 6 g protein, 35 g carbohydrates, 1 g sugar, 5 g total fat, 19% calories from fat, 4 g fiber, 279 mg sodium

PIZZA CRUST

MAKES 4 SERVINGS (2 PIZZAS, ABOUT 9" EACH)

Here's how to make an easy, oil-free, delicious pizza crust at home.

1½ cups warm water

2 packets (about 5 teaspoons) quick-rise yeast (see Yeast Note)

1 tablespoon coconut sugar

4 cups all-purpose white wheat flour (see Flour Note)

¾ teaspoon sea salt

In a small bowl, combine the warm water, yeast, and sugar. (Hot water will kill the yeast and cold water will not activate it.) Whisk well, and let stand for about 5 minutes, until foamy. Meanwhile, in a large bowl, combine the flour and salt. Stir. Add the yeast and water to the flour. Use a large spoon to stir the mixture together. Once the dough comes together, lightly flour the countertop, transfer the dough to it, and begin to knead it. (You can also knead the dough right inside the bowl.) Knead for just a couple of minutes. Coat a large bowl with cooking spray and transfer the dough to that bowl. Cover the bowl with plastic wrap. Place it on a countertop in a warm but not hot area, to let the dough rest and rise for 30 minutes or more, until doubled in size.

Preheat the oven to 500°F for at least 45 minutes. Lightly coat two large pieces of parchment with cooking spray. Divide the dough into two pieces. Transfer each half to parchment, and use your fingers to shape the dough into crusts. (There's no need to make them perfectly round.)

YEAST NOTE • You can use standard baking yeast, if you prefer. If you do, give the dough more time to rise—at least 1½ hours.

FLOUR NOTE • White flour gives a soft, light texture, but you can also substitute whole wheat pastry flour, if you prefer.

(continued)

Add toppings to the pizza (see Pizza! Pizza!). Use a large plate to transfer the pizza (still on the parchment) to a baking sheet or pizza stone. Bake for 10 to 12 minutes, until the crust is golden and crispy on the bottom and the toppings are heated through. Remove, let cool enough to cut into slices (about 5 minutes), and serve.

Shown in color insert pages

NUTRITIONAL FACTS
Per serving: 432 calories, 17 g protein, 91 g carbohydrates, 4 g sugar, 3 g total fat, 6% calories from fat, 14 g fiber, 446 mg sodium

PIZZA! PIZZA!

MAKES 4 SERVINGS (2 PIZZAS)

It's easy and fun to throw your own pizza party at home! You can mix up the toppings, but here's a recipe to get you started.

1 batch Pizza Crust (page 145)

1–1½ cups jarred pasta sauce, tomato sauce, or pizza sauce of choice

1½ cups chopped artichoke hearts (frozen or canned, not marinated in oil)

1 cup chopped red or green bell pepper

½ cup chopped sun-dried tomatoes

½ cup sliced kalamata or green olives

Mushroom "Bacon" Topper (page 181) or an additional 1 cup bell peppers (optional)

½ cup sliced green onion or chopped onion (optional)

½ cup julienned fresh basil (optional)

2 tablespoons Balsamic Drizzle (page 83; optional)

Prepare the pizza crust and preheat the oven to 500°F.

Spread the sauce evenly over both crusts. Distribute the artichoke hearts, peppers, sun-dried tomatoes, olives, Mushroom "Bacon" Topper or additional peppers, and onions (if using) over the pizza crusts. Use a large plate to transfer the pizza (still on the parchment) to a baking sheet or pizza stone. Bake for 10 to 12 minutes, or until the crust is golden and crispy on the bottom and the toppings are heated through. Let the pizza cool enough to cut into slices (about 5 minutes), and serve topped with fresh basil (if using) and the Balsamic Drizzle (if using).

Shown in color insert pages

NUTRITIONAL FACTS

Per serving: 549 calories, 21 g protein, 112 g carbohydrates, 13 g sugar, 7 g total fat, 11% calories from fat, 22 g fiber, 1,121 mg sodium

SCALLOPED POTATO DUO

MAKES 5 SERVINGS

Everyone loves scalloped potatoes, and the combination of white and sweet potatoes makes this recipe a major hit.

Potato Base

- ¾ cup cannellini or other white beans
- ½ cup sliced white portion of green onions or ⅓ cup chopped shallots or onion
- 1 tablespoon nutritional yeast
- 2 teaspoons Dijon mustard
- 1 teaspoon sea salt
- ½ teaspoon dried rosemary or 1 teaspoon chopped fresh rosemary
- ⅛ teaspoon freshly grated nutmeg
- 1 small clove garlic
- 2¼ cups plain low-fat nondairy milk
- 1½ tablespoons freshly squeezed lemon juice
- 1½ tablespoons tahini
  Freshly ground black pepper to taste (optional)
- 1–1¼ pounds Yukon or red potatoes, thinly sliced, peeling optional (see Potatoes Note)
- 1–1¼ pounds sweet potatoes, peeled

Topping

- ½ cup good-quality breadcrumbs (see Toppings Note)
- ½ tablespoon nutritional yeast
  Pinch of sea salt

To make the potato base: In a blender, combine the beans, onions, yeast, mustard, salt, rosemary, nutmeg, garlic, milk, lemon juice, tahini, and pepper (if using). Puree until very smooth.

Preheat the oven to 400°F. Line a baking sheet with parchment paper and place it on a lower rack to catch any possible drippings. Use cooking spray to lightly coat the bottom and sides of an 8" x 12" casserole dish.

Add one-quarter of the sauce to the prepared dish to cover the bottom with a thin layer. Add a layer of white or red potatoes (about half of the total amount) to the dish, followed by a layer of about one-quarter of the sauce. (The layers do not need to be completely even or measured out; it just helps to layer the potatoes with the sauce a few times to get it between some of the potatoes.) Repeat the process, creating a layer of all the sweet potatoes, then finish with the remaining white or red potatoes covered with the remaining sauce.

To make the topping: In a small bowl, combine the breadcrumbs, yeast, and salt. Sprinkle the mixture over the top of the potatoes and sauce, and cover with aluminum foil. Bake for 50 to 60 minutes, or until the potatoes are cooked through. Remove the foil and bake for another 5 to 6 minutes, or until lightly browned. (You can also set the oven to broil for just a minute to get that golden color on top.) Let sit for 5 to 10 minutes before serving.

POTATOES NOTE • You can vary the proportions to suit your own tastes. For a "saucier" casserole, use only 2 pounds of potatoes.

TOPPINGS NOTE • Almond meal is a very tasty, gluten-free substitution. You can use ¼ cup in place of the ½ cup of breadcrumbs, or use equal amounts of each (¼ cup almond meal and ¼ cup crumbs).

NUTRITIONAL FACTS
Per serving: 266 calories, 11 g protein, 48 g carbohydrates, 9 g sugar, 4 g total fat, 14% calories from fat, 7 g fiber, 806 mg sodium

BBQ LENTILS

MAKES 5 SERVINGS

The seasonings lend a light barbecue flavor to these easy-to-prepare lentils.

2 cups dried green or brown lentils, rinsed

3 tablespoons balsamic vinegar

4½ cups water

½ cup tomato paste

2 tablespoons vegan Worcestershire sauce

2 teaspoons dried rosemary

1 teaspoon onion powder

½ teaspoon garlic powder

½ teaspoon allspice

¼ teaspoon sea salt

1 tablespoon coconut nectar or pure maple syrup

In a large saucepan over medium-high heat, combine the lentils with 2 tablespoons of the vinegar. Cook, stirring, for 5 to 7 minutes to lightly toast the lentils. Once the pan is getting dry, add the water, tomato paste, Worcestershire sauce, rosemary, onion powder, garlic powder, allspice, salt, nectar or syrup, and the remaining 1 tablespoon vinegar, and stir through. Bring to a boil, then reduce the heat to low, cover the pot, and cook for 37 to 40 minutes, or until the lentils are fully tender. Season to taste, and serve.

NUTRITIONAL FACTS
Per serving: 295 calories, 20 g protein, 54 g carbohydrates, 9 g sugar, 1 g total fat, 3% calories from fat, 14 g fiber, 399 mg sodium

PRESSURE-STEWED CHICKPEAS

MAKES 5 SERVINGS

This recipe can be prepared on the stovetop or in an instant pot. The onions and dates turn into a smoky-sweet saucy base, developing wonderful flavors.

- 3 tablespoons water
- 2 large or 3 small to medium onions, chopped (3–3½ cups)
- 1½ tablespoons smoked paprika
- ½ teaspoon ground cumin
- ⅛–¼ teaspoon ground allspice

- Rounded ½ teaspoon sea salt
- 2 cans (15 ounces each) chickpeas, rinsed and drained
- ⅔ cup chopped, pitted dates
- 1 jar (24 ounces) strained tomatoes (see Note)

In the instant pot set on the sauté function, combine the water, onions, paprika, cumin, allspice, and salt. Cook for 6 to 7 minutes, stirring occasionally. If the mixture is sticking, add another tablespoon or two of water. Add the chickpeas, dates, and tomatoes, and stir well. Turn off the sauté function, and put on the lid. Manually set to pressure cook on high for 18 minutes. Release the pressure or let the pressure release naturally. Stir, taste, season as desired, and serve.

STOVETOP METHOD: If you don't have an instant pot, simply use a large pot and cook on the stovetop. Sauté the water, onions, paprika, cumin, allspice, and salt. After adding the chickpeas, dates, and tomatoes, bring to a boil, then reduce the heat to low. Cover and cook for 40 minutes, or until the dates and onions have softened.

NOTE • If you're unable to find strained tomatoes, you can substitute a 28-ounce can of crushed tomatoes.

SERVING IDEA: Serve with cooked rice, quinoa, or other whole grain.

NUTRITIONAL FACTS
Per serving: 258 calories, 10 g protein, 50 g carbohydrates, 23 g sugar, 4 g total fat, 12% calories from fat, 13 g fiber, 742 mg sodium

POWER PASTA

MAKES 4 SERVINGS

Power up your favorite pasta sauce! Lentils make the sauce heartier and more nutritious.

⅔ cup dried red lentils

1½ cups water

1–1½ cups sliced or chopped carrots

½ teaspoon dried rosemary or 1 teaspoon dried basil

½ teaspoon fennel seed

1 pound dry pasta

1 jar (24 ounces) pasta sauce of choice

Couple pinches of sea salt (see Note)

1 teaspoon pure maple syrup (optional)

5–6 cups baby spinach leaves (optional)

In a large pot, boil water for the pasta. Meanwhile, in a medium pot, combine the lentils, water, carrots, rosemary or basil, and fennel. Bring to a boil over high heat. Reduce the heat to low, cover, and let cook for 10 to 15 minutes, or until the lentils are fully cooked and soft.

Once the lentils are almost cooked through, cook the pasta. Mash or lightly puree the lentil mixture using an immersion blender, if a smoother texture is desired. Add the pasta sauce to the lentils, and gently heat through over low to medium heat. Taste, and add the salt and syrup (if using). Add the spinach (if using) and stir until just wilted. Drain the pasta and serve in bowls topped with the lentil sauce.

NOTE • Jarred pasta sauces vary in sodium and flavor. Start with a couple pinches of salt, and add more to taste if needed.

NUTRITIONAL FACTS
Per serving: 730 calories, 29 g protein, 138 g carbohydrates, 18 g sugar, 7 g total fat, 9% calories from fat, 15 g fiber, 889 mg sodium

THAI RED LENTILS

MAKES 4 SERVINGS

This recipe is simple to prepare, and yet so satisfying!

2 cups dried red lentils

1 can (13½ ounces) lite coconut milk

2 tablespoons red or yellow Thai curry paste (see Note)

¼–½ teaspoon sea salt (use less if using more curry paste)

2–2¼ cups water

⅓ cup finely chopped fresh basil

3–4 tablespoons lime juice

In a large saucepan over high heat, combine the lentils, coconut milk, curry paste, salt, and 2 cups of the water. Stir and bring to a boil. Reduce the heat to low, cover, and cook for 20 minutes, or until the lentils are fully softened. Add the basil and 3 tablespoons of the lime juice, and stir. Season to taste with more salt and the remaining 1 tablespoon lime juice, if desired. Add the remaining ¼ cup water to thin, if desired.

SERVING IDEAS: Serve straight up in bowls with whole grain pitas for dipping, or use it to top cooked brown rice, quinoa, or another whole grain.

NOTE • Start with 2 tablespoons, and if you enjoy a little more heat and flavor, feel free to add another ½ to 1 tablespoon. For extra heat, you can also add hot sauce to taste.

NUTRITIONAL FACTS

Per serving: 389 calories, 25 g protein, 58 g carbohydrates, 4 g sugar, 8 g total fat, 18% calories from fat, 16 g fiber, 441 mg sodium

SWEET POTATO SHEPHERD'S PIE

MAKES 5 SERVINGS

This delicious, nutritious twist on shepherd's pie is made from a base of lentils and mushrooms with savory seasonings and crowned with a crisp sweet potato topping. Yum!

Filling

- 2 tablespoons red wine
- 1 teaspoon dried thyme
- ½ teaspoon dried rosemary
- ½ teaspoon garlic powder
- 1 pound white button or cremini mushrooms (about 3 cups) or 2 cups minced cauliflower
- 1 cup finely chopped onion
- ½ cup finely chopped carrots
- ½ cup finely chopped celery
- 2 tablespoons whole wheat pastry flour
- 3½ tablespoons tamari
- 1 teaspoon vegan Worcestershire sauce (optional)
- 2 tablespoons tomato paste
- 1 cup water
- 2½ cups cooked lentils
- ½–¾ cup frozen peas

Topping

- 2 cups cubed cooked sweet potato
- 2 teaspoons reduced-sodium tamari
- 1 teaspoon chopped fresh thyme leaves

  Few pinches of freshly grated nutmeg

  Freshly ground black pepper (optional)
- ⅓ cup breadcrumbs

  Pinch of sea salt

To make the filling: In a large pot over high heat, combine the wine, thyme, rosemary, garlic powder, and mushrooms or cauliflower. Cook for 7 to 8 minutes, or until the mushrooms release their juices and begin to reduce down. Add the onion, carrots, and celery, and cook for another 3 to 4 minutes. Add the flour, tamari, and Worcestershire sauce. Reduce the heat to medium-high for a few minutes to cook out the raw flavor of the flour. Stir in the tomato paste and add a few tablespoons of the water. As the mixture thickens, add another ¼ cup or so of the water. Stir, and as the mixture thickens again, add the lentils and the remaining water, and continue to stir. Let it thicken and bubble, then remove the pot from the heat. Stir in the peas. Transfer the mixture to an 8" x 8" baking dish.

To make the topping: Preheat the oven to 400°F. In a medium bowl, mash the sweet potatoes with the tamari, thyme, nutmeg, and pepper (if using). Smooth the sweet potatoes over the filling, using a spatula. Sprinkle on the bread-crumbs and salt on top. Bake for 20 to 25 minutes, until browning around the edges and bubbly. Let it sit for 5 minutes or so, then serve.

NUTRITIONAL FACTS
Per serving: 283 calories, 16 g protein, 54 g carbohydrates, 10 g sugar, 2 g total fat, 5% calories from fat, 12 g fiber, 845 mg sodium

SUN-DRIED PUMPKIN PESTO PASTA WITH FRESH SPINACH

MAKES 4 SERVINGS

This pesto is superb. Try it with any pasta shape you like!

- 1 cup sliced sun-dried tomatoes (see Note)
- 1 large clove garlic, quartered (use 2 if you love a punch of garlic)
- 2 pitted dates
- ¼ teaspoon sea salt
- Freshly ground black pepper to taste (optional)
- ½ cup water

- 2 tablespoons pumpkin seeds or chopped almonds (toast ahead of time if you want more flavor)
- ½ cup fresh parsley leaves
- 1 cup fresh basil leaves + handful of fresh basil leaves, julienned or chopped (optional)
- 1 pound dry pasta of choice
- 3–4 cups fresh baby spinach leaves

In a food processor, combine the sun-dried tomatoes, garlic, dates, salt, and pepper (if using). Pulse to combine. Add the water and puree, scraping down the sides of the bowl as needed. Add the pumpkin seeds or almonds, parsley, and 1 cup of the basil, and pulse several times to incorporate, but keep some texture.

Cook the pasta according to package directions. Once the pasta is almost done, remove ¼ cup of the pasta water and reserve. Drain the pasta (do not rinse), and return it to the pot. Place over very low heat. Add the pesto and spinach leaves, and gently work the pesto through the pasta. If the pasta seems dry, add some of the reserved cooking water, a couple tablespoons at a time, until the sauce reaches the desired consistency. Once the spinach is just wilted, taste, and add extra salt if desired. Garnish with the handful of fresh basil (if using) before serving.

NOTE • Sun-dried tomatoes can be purchased dry-packed or in oil. If purchasing dry, the flavor is optimal, however they can be tough and chewy. So before processing, soak them in ½ to 1 cup of boiled or hot water for about 10 minutes. Don't discard that water; keep it for the puree, as it is flavorful. Oil-packed tomatoes are easier to find, but you will need to fully drain and then rinse them well with hot water. This helps remove not only the oil but also some of the marinated flavors that aren't very fresh-tasting.

NUTRITIONAL FACTS
Per serving: 569 calories, 22 g protein, 109 g carbohydrates, 9 g sugar, 5 g total fat, 8% calories from fat, 9 g fiber, 452 mg sodium

PASTA CARBONARA

MAKES 4 SERVINGS

This dish is luscious and rich, and the black salt lends the characteristic "eggy" flavor. It's also delicious served with Mushroom "Bacon" Topper (page 181).

2 cups steamed cauliflower florets

⅓ cup soaked and drained raw cashews

1½ tablespoons chickpea miso (or other mild-flavored miso)

1–2 large cloves garlic (see Note)

½ teaspoon sea salt

½ teaspoon black salt

1½ cups plain low-fat nondairy milk

2 tablespoons lemon juice

Few pinches of freshly grated nutmeg and/or black pepper

1 pound dry pasta

½–¾ cup frozen peas (optional)

¼–⅓ cup water

Boil the water for the pasta. Meanwhile, in a blender, combine the cauliflower, cashews, miso, garlic, sea salt, black salt, milk, lemon juice, and nutmeg and/or pepper. Puree until very smooth. Prepare the pasta according to package directions. Once the pasta is almost cooked (still having some "bite," not mushy), add the peas to the cooking water and then immediately drain, and return the pasta and peas to the pot. Pour the sauce from the blender into the pot. Use the water to swish and rinse any remaining sauce from the blender into the pot. Gently heat the pasta and sauce over medium-low heat for a minute or two, or until the sauce thickens. Taste, and add additional salt and pepper if desired.

NOTE • The garlic will not be sautéed or otherwise cooked in advance to soften the flavor, so be a little judicious in how much you use. If you have young children, they may not enjoy the sauce with a lot of garlic. If you love garlic, feel free to use the two large cloves—or more.

NUTRITIONAL FACTS
Per serving: 616 calories, 24 g protein, 110 g carbohydrates, 7 g sugar, 9 g total fat, 12% calories from fat, 8 g fiber, 875 mg sodium

ORANGE TOFU

MAKES 4 SERVINGS

This tofu is baked in the oven in a lightly sweetened orange and tahini sauce. Try serving it over Coconut Curry Rice (page 184).

⅓ cup freshly squeezed orange juice (zest orange first; see below)

1 tablespoon tamari

1 tablespoon tahini

½ tablespoon coconut nectar or pure maple syrup

2 tablespoons apple cider vinegar

½ tablespoon freshly grated ginger

1 large clove garlic, grated

½–1 teaspoon orange zest

¼ teaspoon sea salt

Few pinches of crushed red-pepper flakes (optional)

1 package (12 ounces) extra-firm tofu, sliced into ¼"–½" thick squares and patted to remove excess moisture

Preheat the oven to 400°F.

In a small bowl, combine the orange juice, tamari, tahini, nectar or syrup, vinegar, ginger, garlic, orange zest, salt, and red-pepper flakes (if using). Whisk until well combined. Pour the sauce into an 8" x 12" baking dish. Add the tofu and turn to coat both sides. Bake for 20 minutes. Add salt to taste.

SERVING IDEA: Serve over cooked whole grains such as quinoa, brown rice, or whole wheat couscous, or pair with sweet potatoes and steamed greens.

NUTRITIONAL FACTS
Per serving: 122 calories, 10 g protein, 7 g carbohydrates, 4 g sugar, 7 g total fat, 49% calories from fat, 1 g fiber, 410 mg sodium

SOUTHWEST TOFU

MAKES 4 SERVINGS

A one-dish tofu recipe with a pop of flavor! Delicious with rice and Salsa Make-over (page 75).

3½ tablespoons freshly squeezed lime juice

2 teaspoons pure maple syrup

1½ teaspoons ground cumin

1 teaspoon dried oregano leaves

1 teaspoon chili powder

½ teaspoon paprika

½ teaspoon sea salt

⅛ teaspoon allspice

1 package (12 ounces) extra-firm tofu, sliced into ¼"–½" thick squares and patted to remove excess moisture

Preheat the oven to 400°F.

In a 9" x 12" baking dish, combine the lime juice, syrup, cumin, oregano, chili powder, paprika, salt, and allspice. Add the tofu and turn to coat both sides. Bake uncovered for 20 minutes, or until the marinade is absorbed, turning once.

SERVING IDEAS: Serve over brown rice, quinoa, or pasta, or serve it cooled in a salad.

NUTRITIONAL FACTS
Per serving: 78 calories, 7 g protein, 6 g carbohydrates, 3 g sugar, 4 g total fat, 42% calories from fat, 1 g fiber, 324 mg sodium

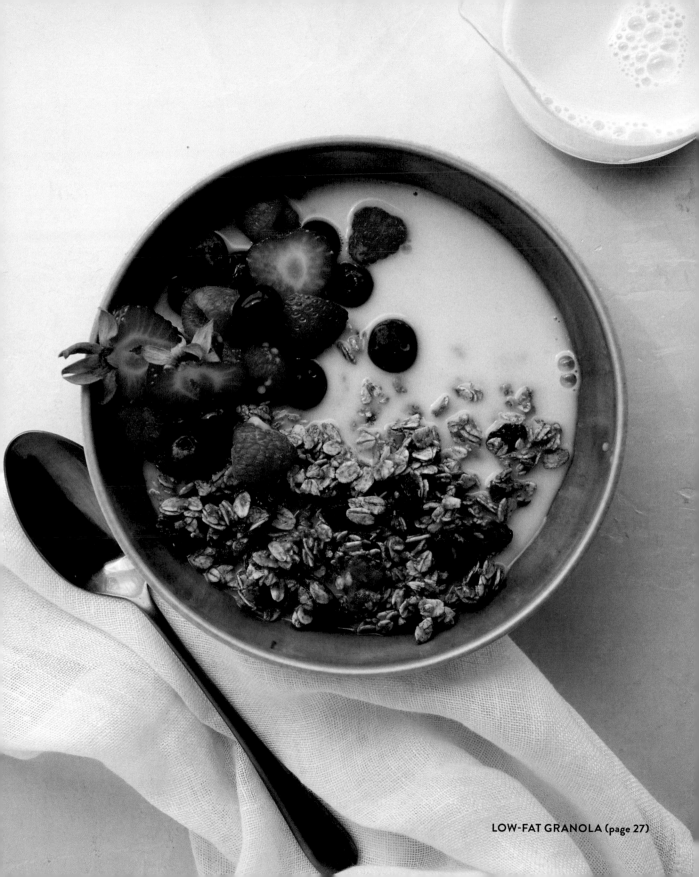

LOW-FAT GRANOLA (page 27)

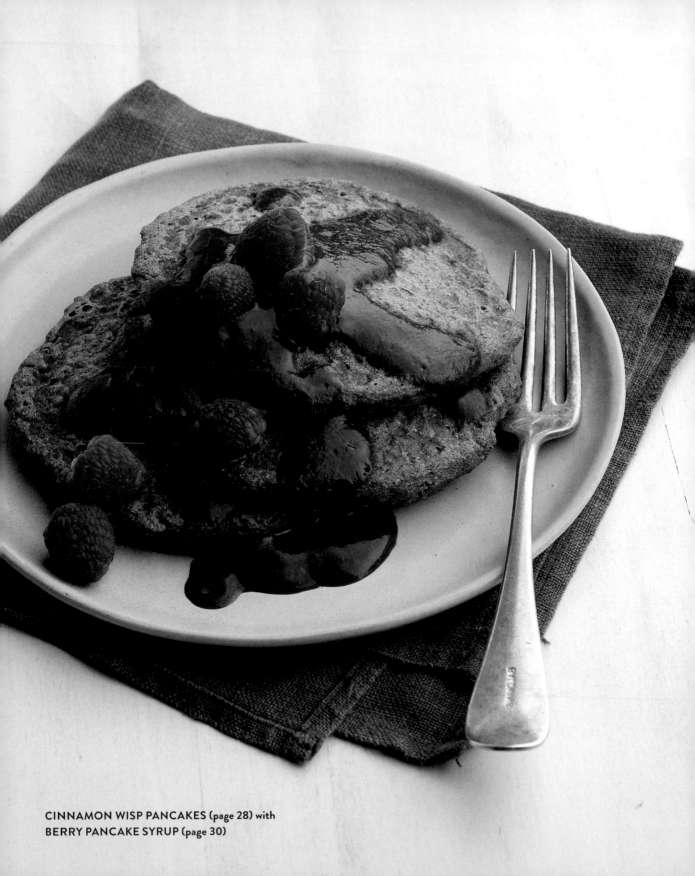

CINNAMON WISP PANCAKES (page 28) with
BERRY PANCAKE SYRUP (page 30)

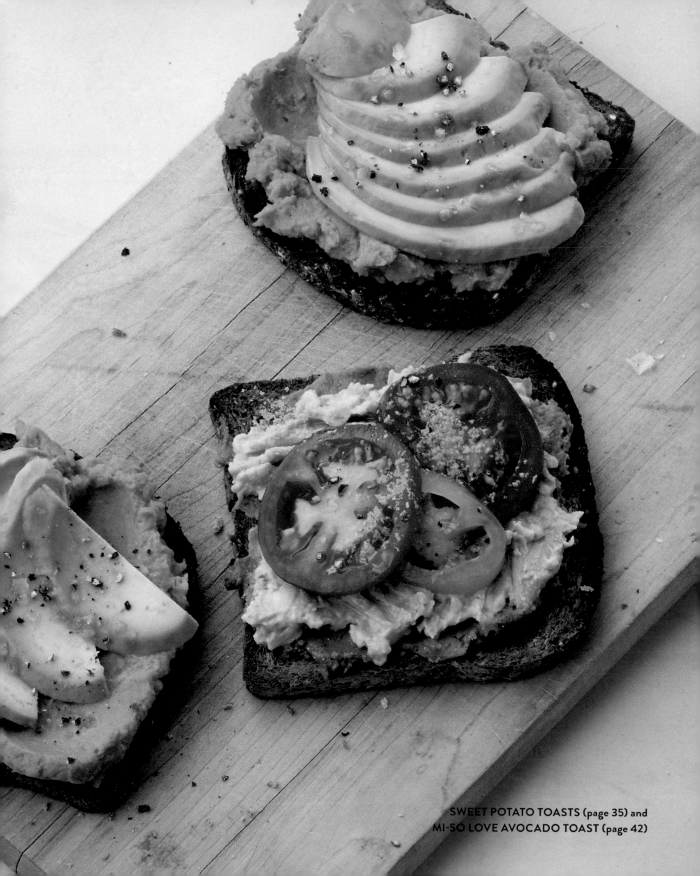

SWEET POTATO TOASTS (page 35) and
MI-SO LOVE AVOCADO TOAST (page 42)

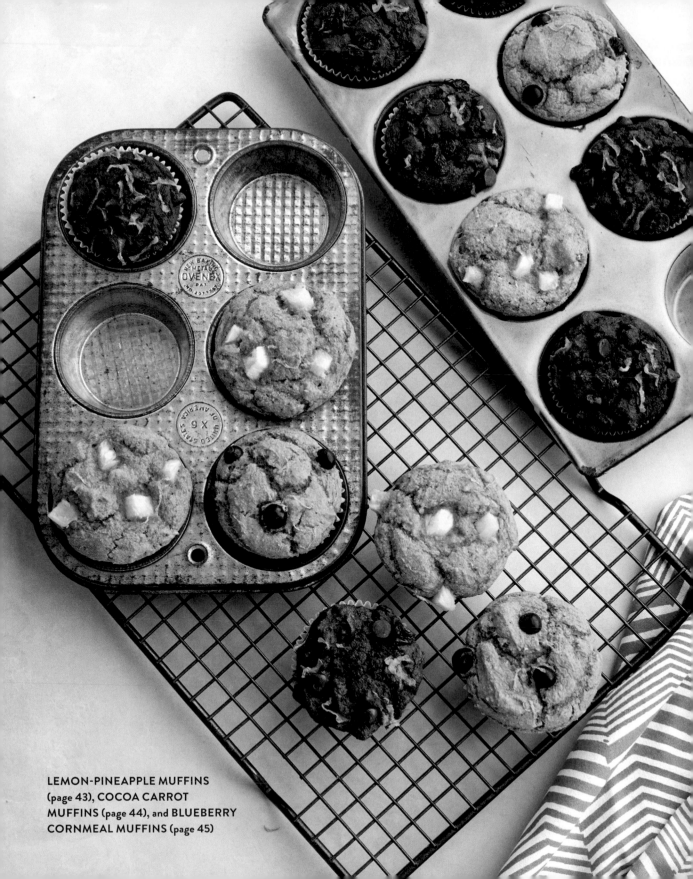

LEMON-PINEAPPLE MUFFINS
(page 43), COCOA CARROT
MUFFINS (page 44), and BLUEBERRY
CORNMEAL MUFFINS (page 45)

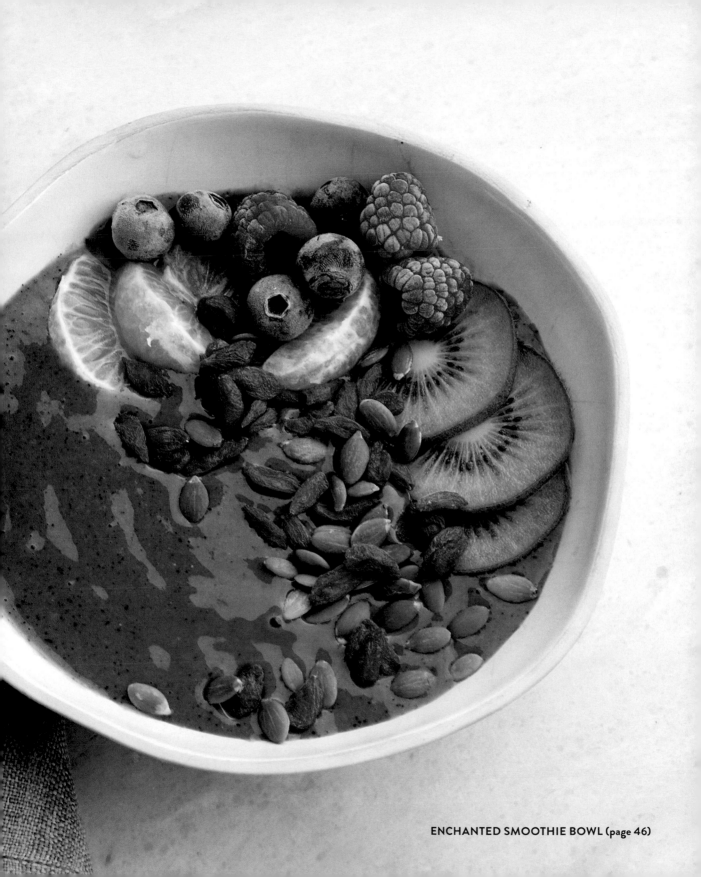

ENCHANTED SMOOTHIE BOWL (page 46)

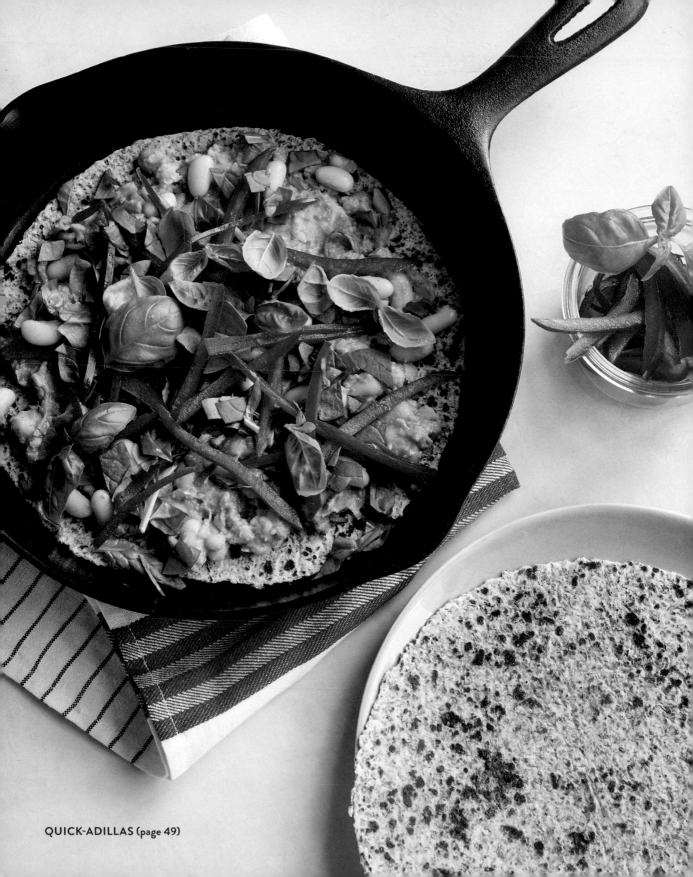

QUICK-ADILLAS (page 49)

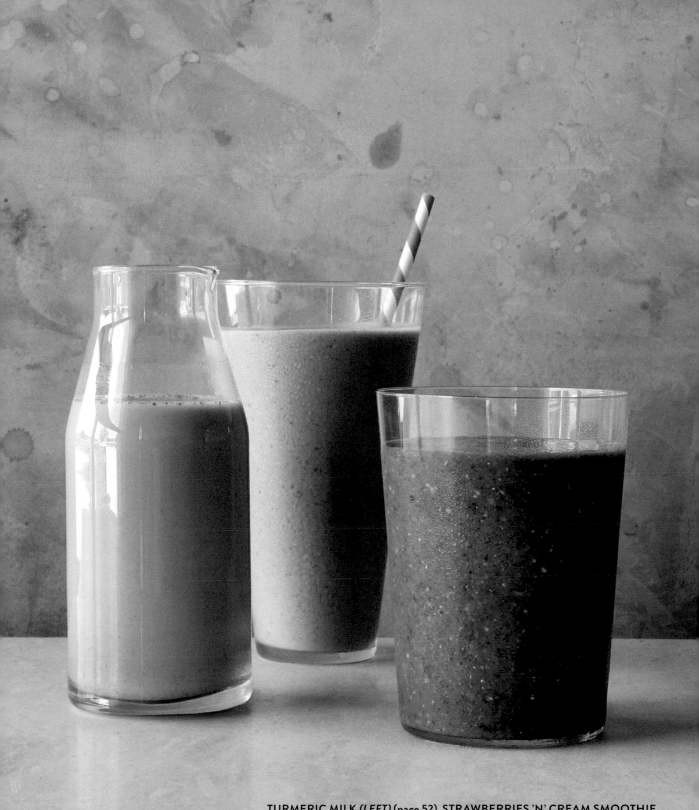

TURMERIC MILK *(LEFT)* (page 52), STRAWBERRIES 'N' CREAM SMOOTHIE *(MIDDLE)* (page 54), and BIG GREEN SMOOTHIE *(RIGHT)* (page 55)

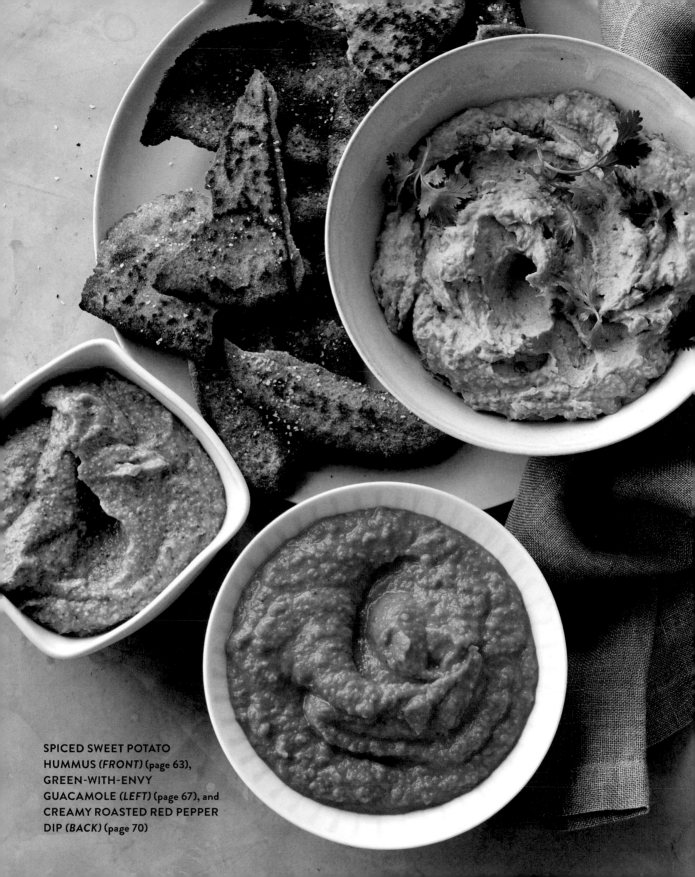

SPICED SWEET POTATO
HUMMUS *(FRONT)* (page 63),
GREEN-WITH-ENVY
GUACAMOLE *(LEFT)* (page 67), and
CREAMY ROASTED RED PEPPER
DIP *(BACK)* (page 70)

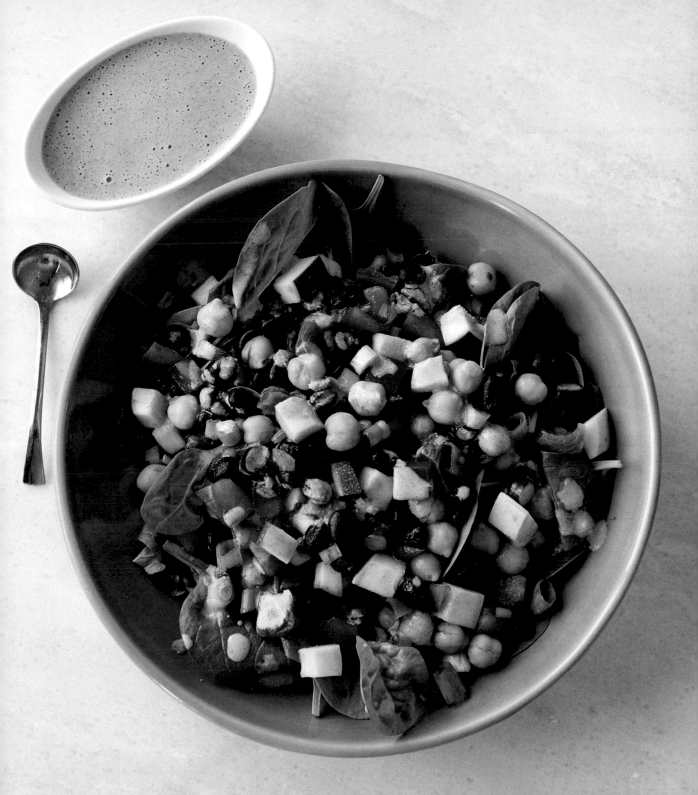

MOROCCAN BEAN SALAD (page 91) with
MOROCCAN SALAD DRESSING (page 90)

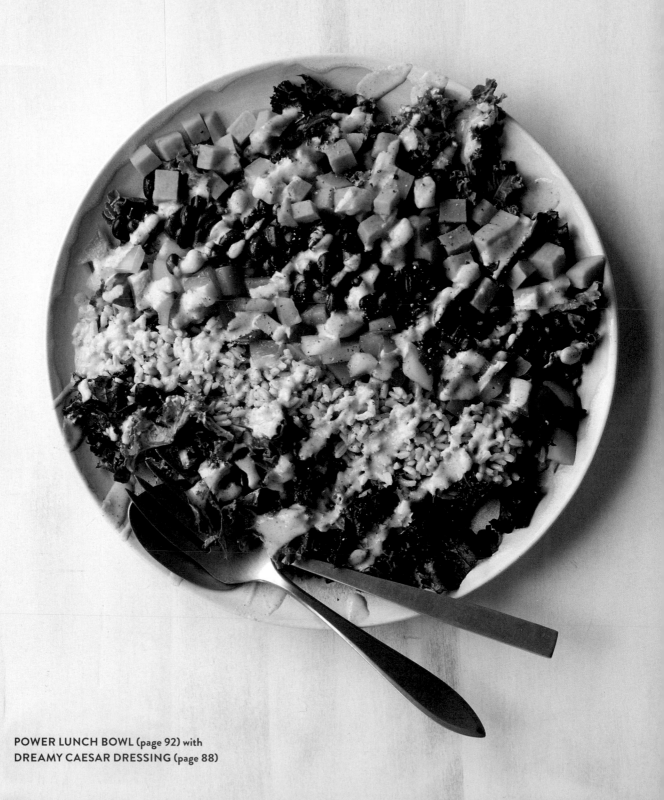

POWER LUNCH BOWL (page 92) with
DREAMY CAESAR DRESSING (page 88)

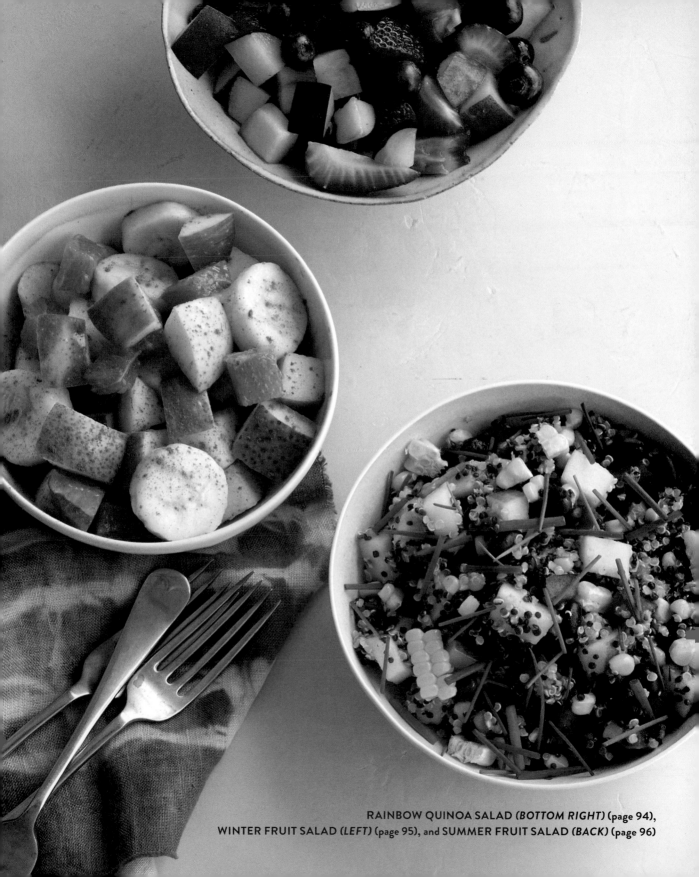

RAINBOW QUINOA SALAD *(BOTTOM RIGHT)* (page 94),
WINTER FRUIT SALAD *(LEFT)* (page 95), and SUMMER FRUIT SALAD *(BACK)* (page 96)

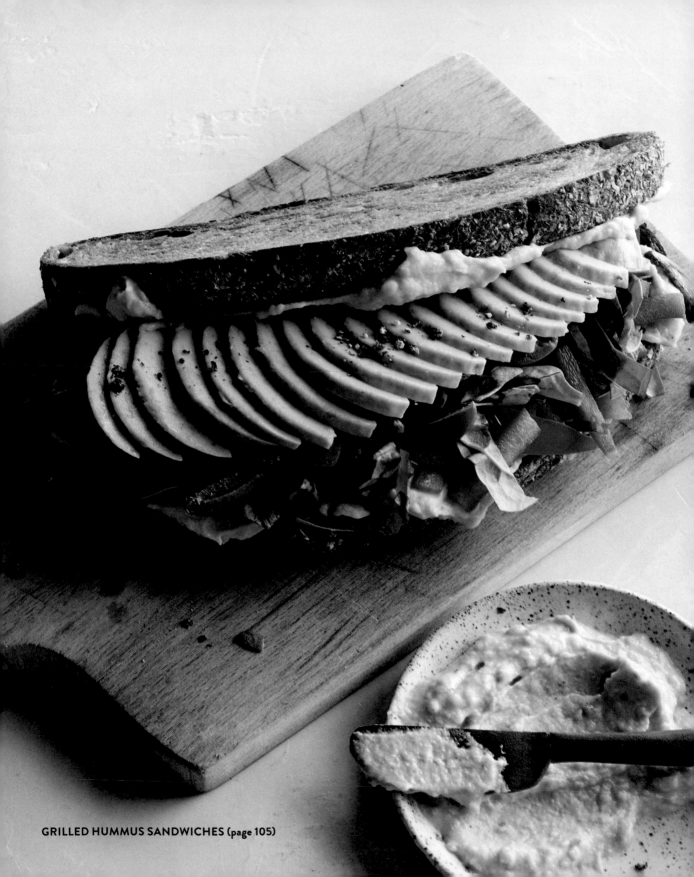

GRILLED HUMMUS SANDWICHES (page 105)

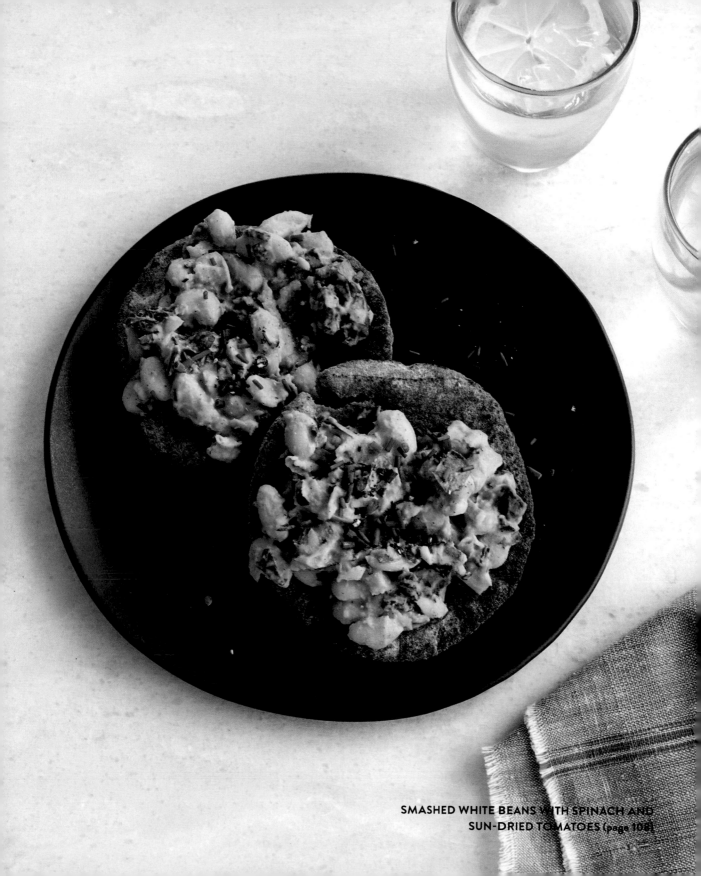

SMASHED WHITE BEANS WITH SPINACH AND
SUN-DRIED TOMATOES (page 108)

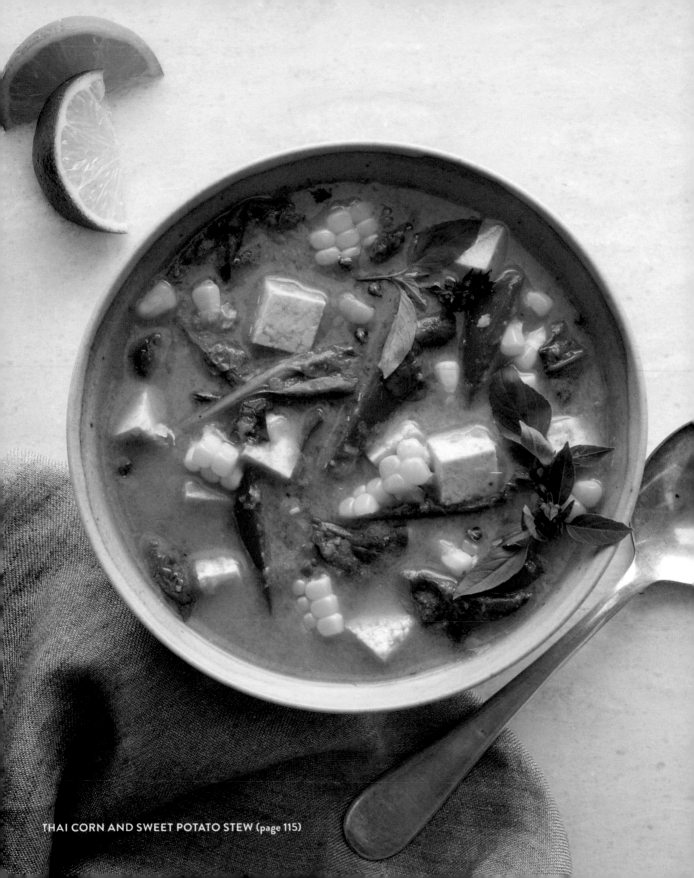

THAI CORN AND SWEET POTATO STEW (page 115)

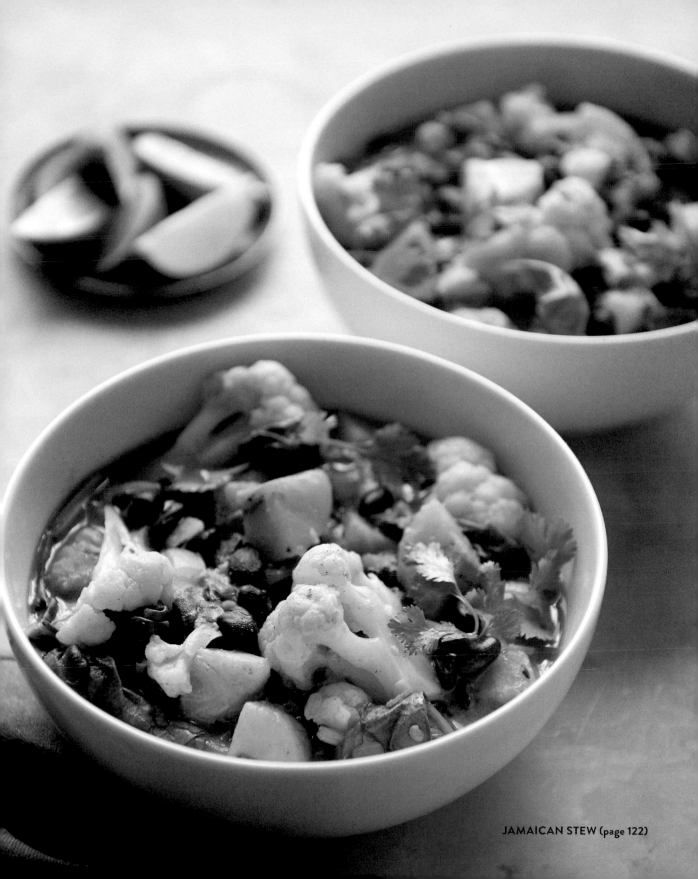

JAMAICAN STEW (page 122)

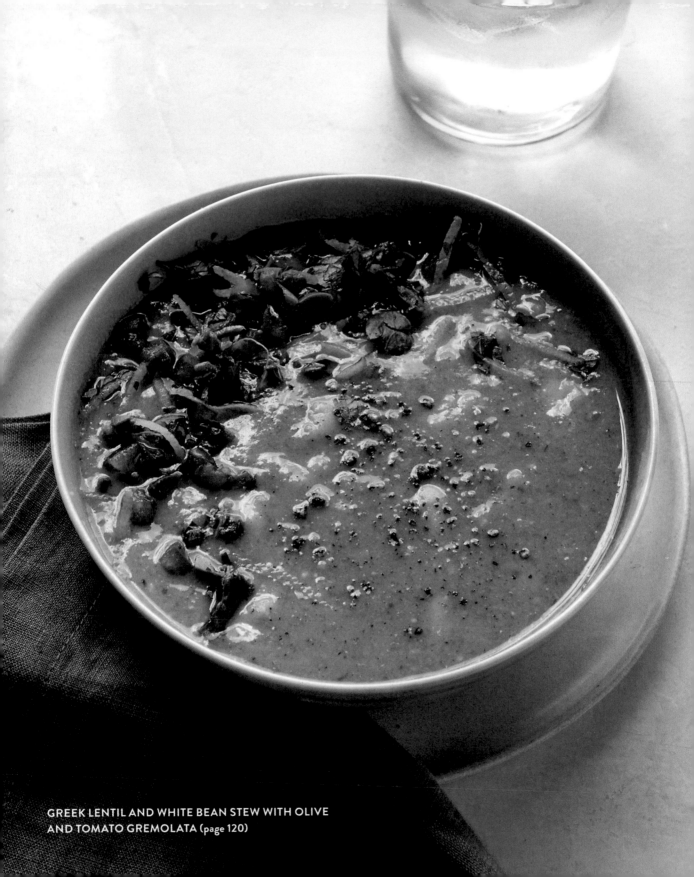

GREEK LENTIL AND WHITE BEAN STEW WITH OLIVE
AND TOMATO GREMOLATA (page 120)

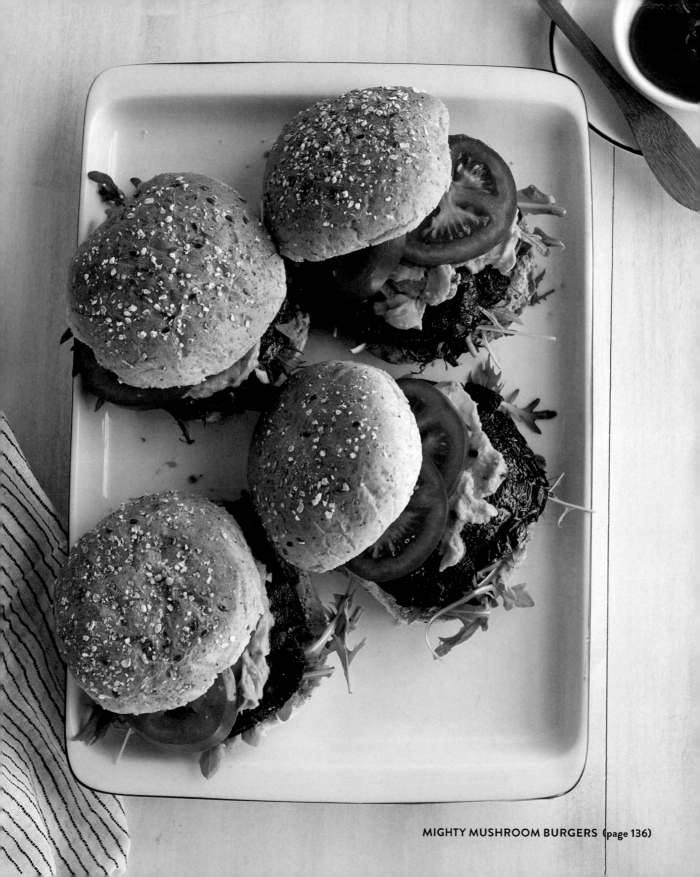

MIGHTY MUSHROOM BURGERS (page 136)

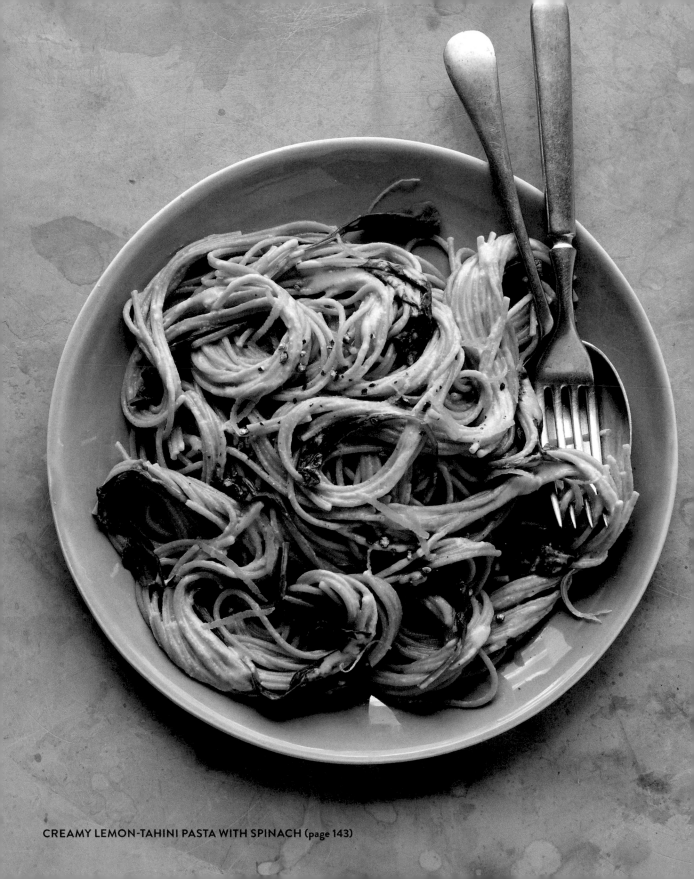

CREAMY LEMON-TAHINI PASTA WITH SPINACH (page 143)

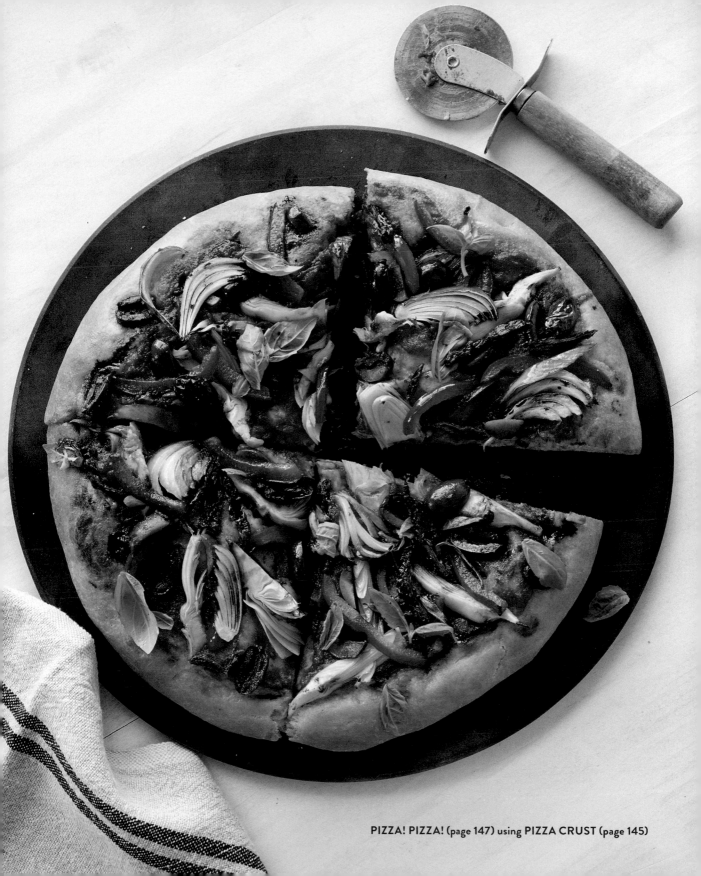

PIZZA! PIZZA! (page 147) using PIZZA CRUST (page 145)

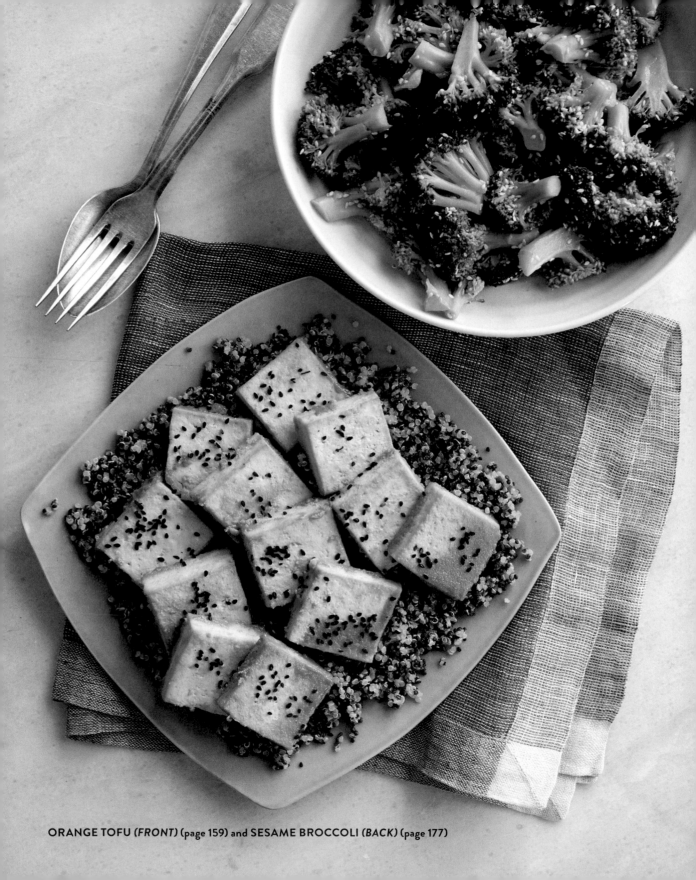

ORANGE TOFU *(FRONT)* (page 159) and SESAME BROCCOLI *(BACK)* (page 177)

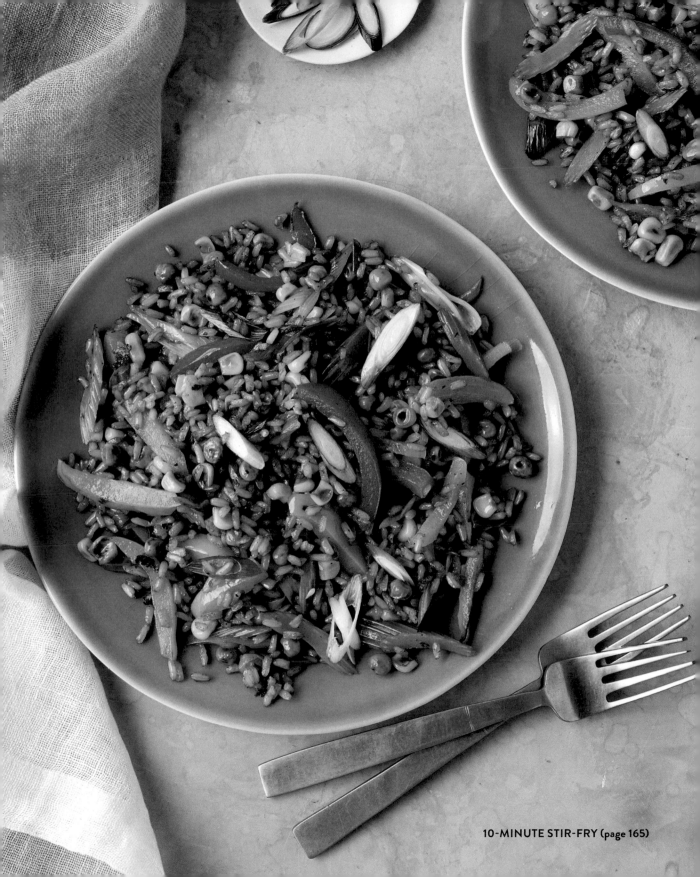

10-MINUTE STIR-FRY (page 165)

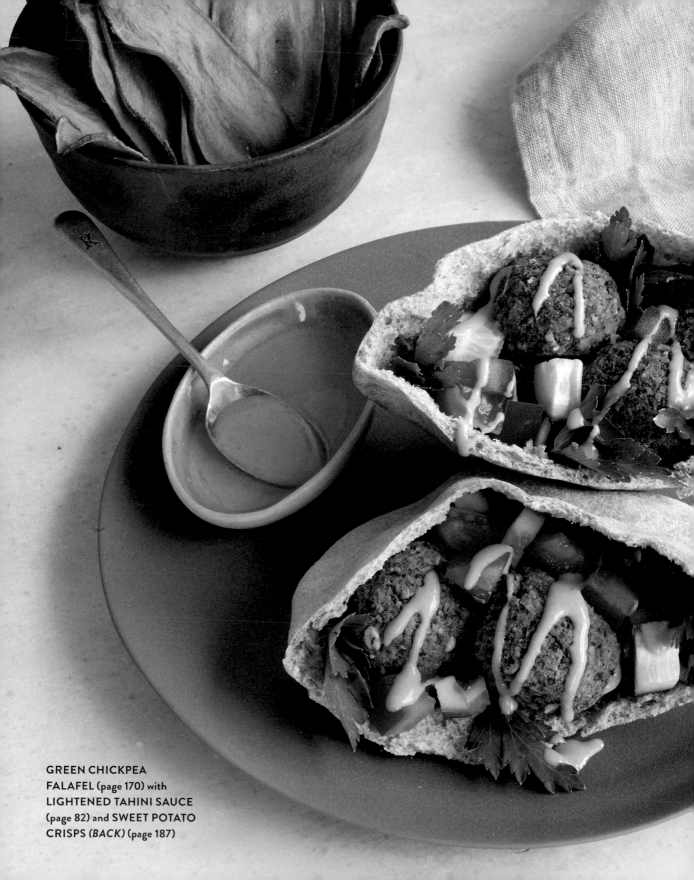

GREEN CHICKPEA
FALAFEL (page 170) with
LIGHTENED TAHINI SAUCE
(page 82) and SWEET POTATO
CRISPS (*BACK*) (page 187)

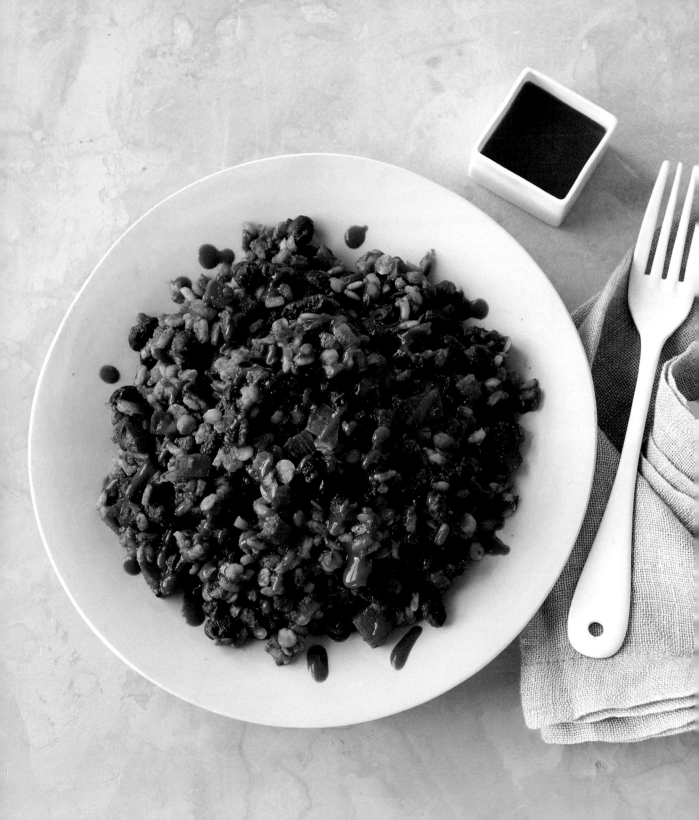

TEX-MEX RICE 'N BEANS (page 168)

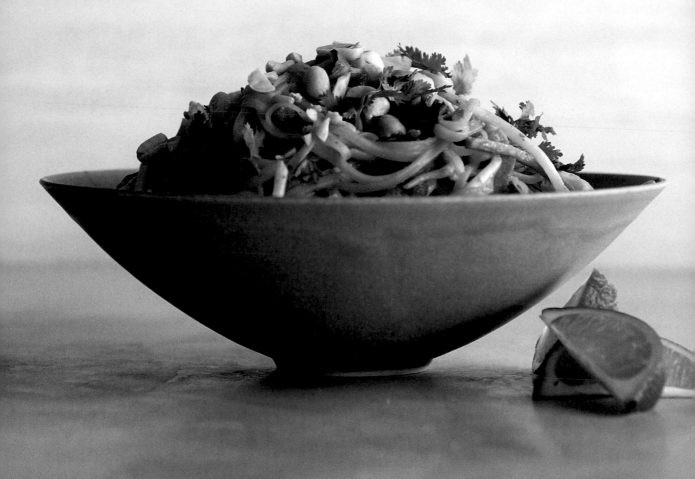

RAD THAI (page 171)

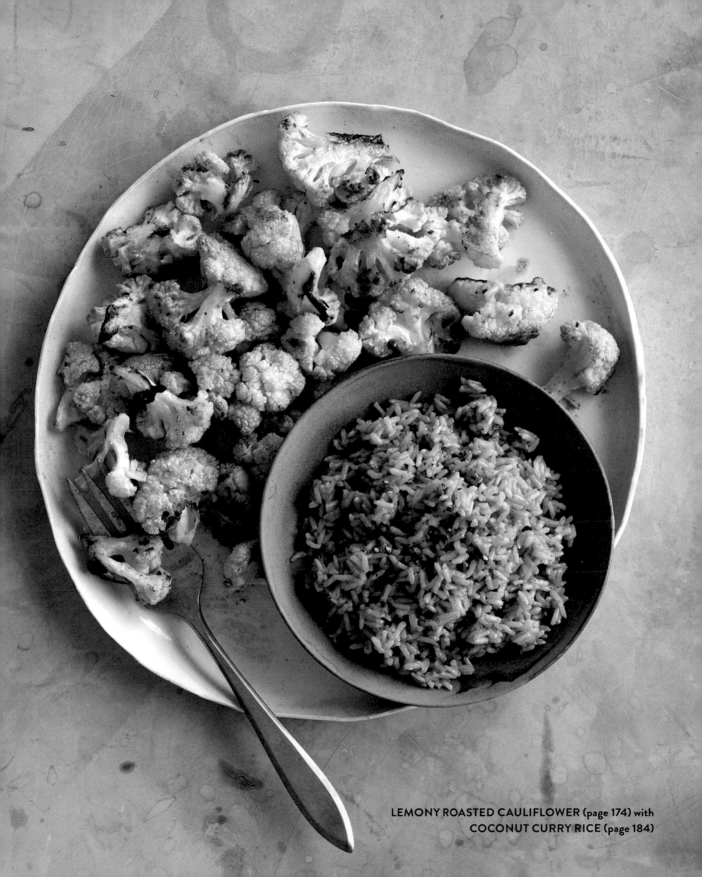

LEMONY ROASTED CAULIFLOWER (page 174) with COCONUT CURRY RICE (page 184)

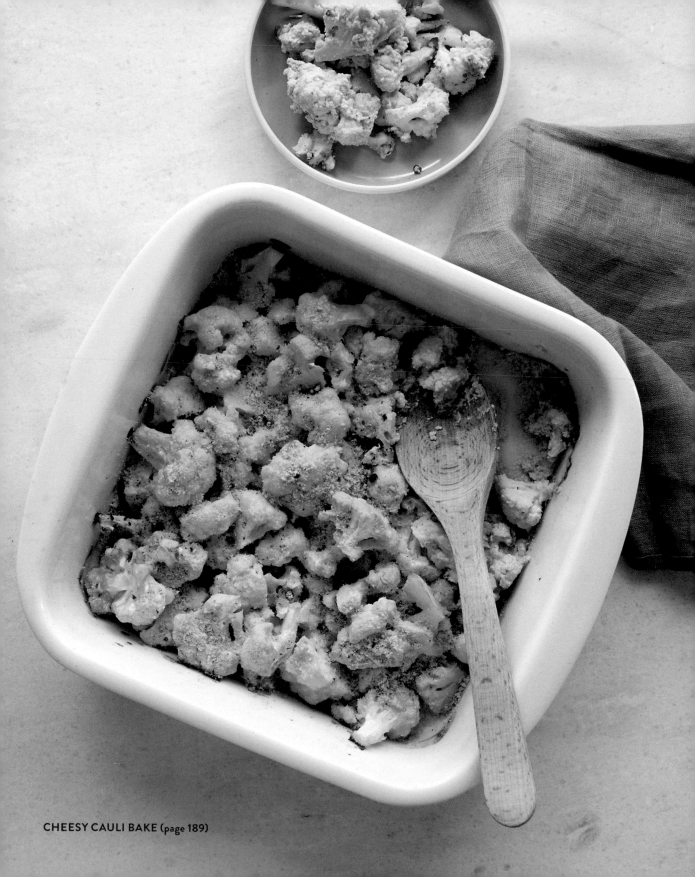

CHEESY CAULI BAKE (page 189)

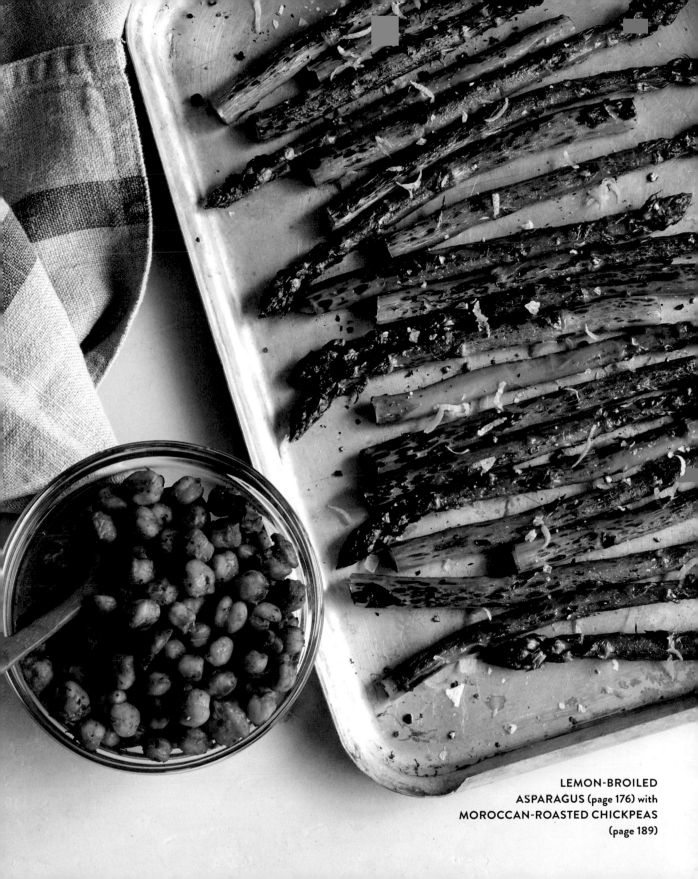

LEMON-BROILED
ASPARAGUS (page 176) with
MOROCCAN-ROASTED CHICKPEAS
(page 189)

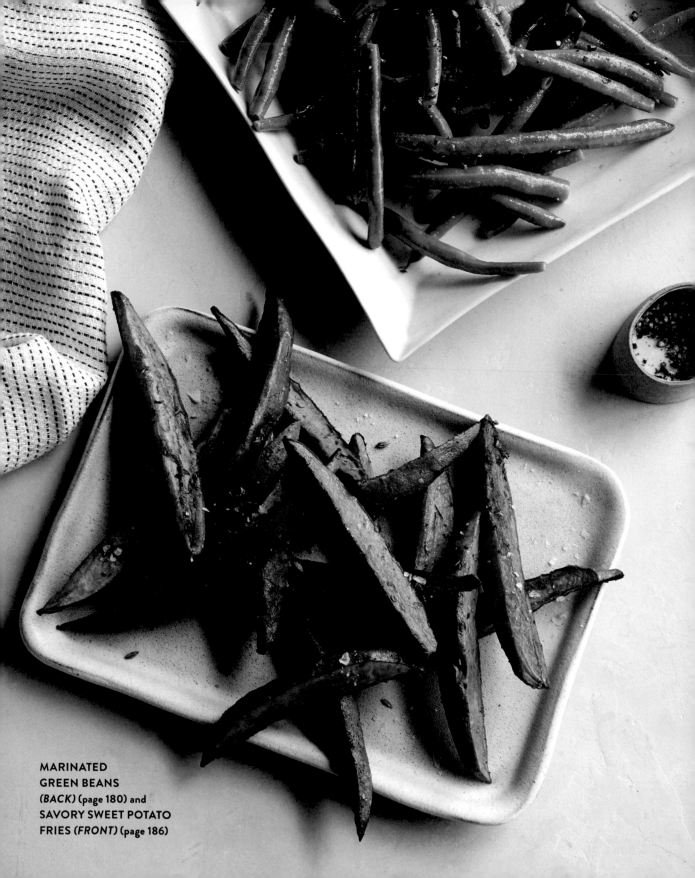

MARINATED
GREEN BEANS
(BACK) (page 180) and
SAVORY SWEET POTATO
FRIES *(FRONT)* (page 186)

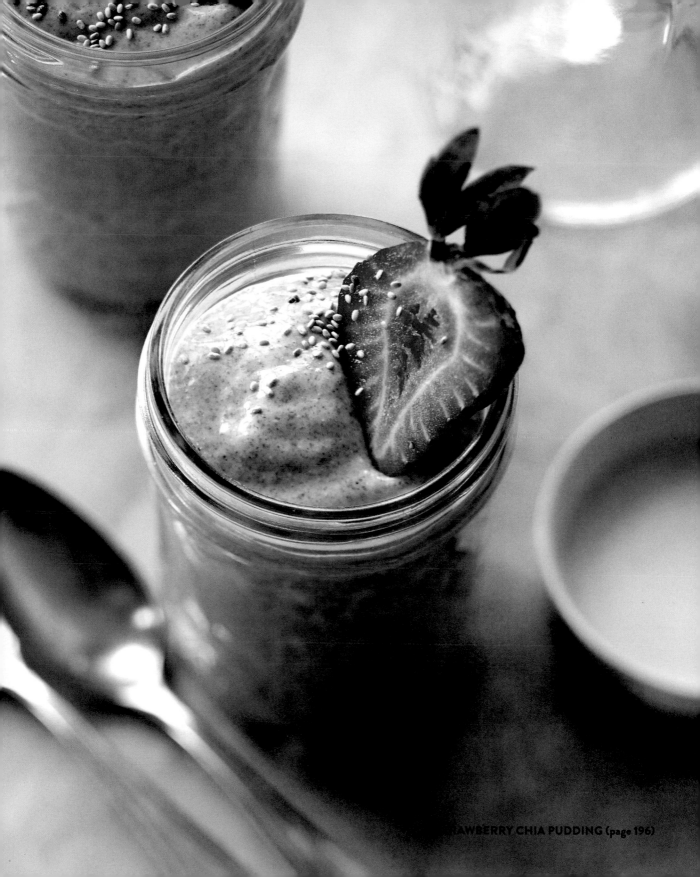

STRAWBERRY CHIA PUDDING (page 196)

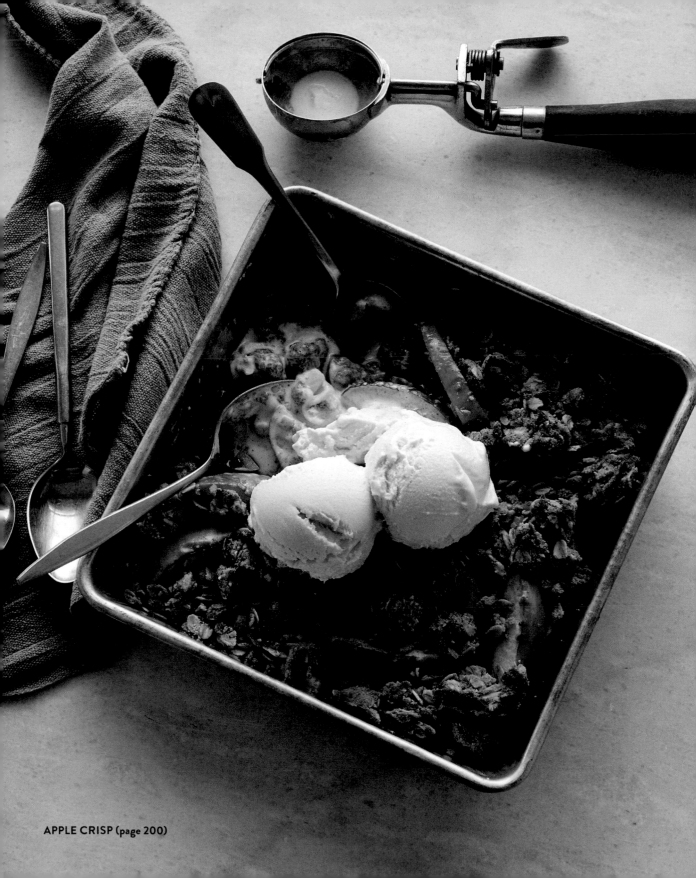

APPLE CRISP (page 200)

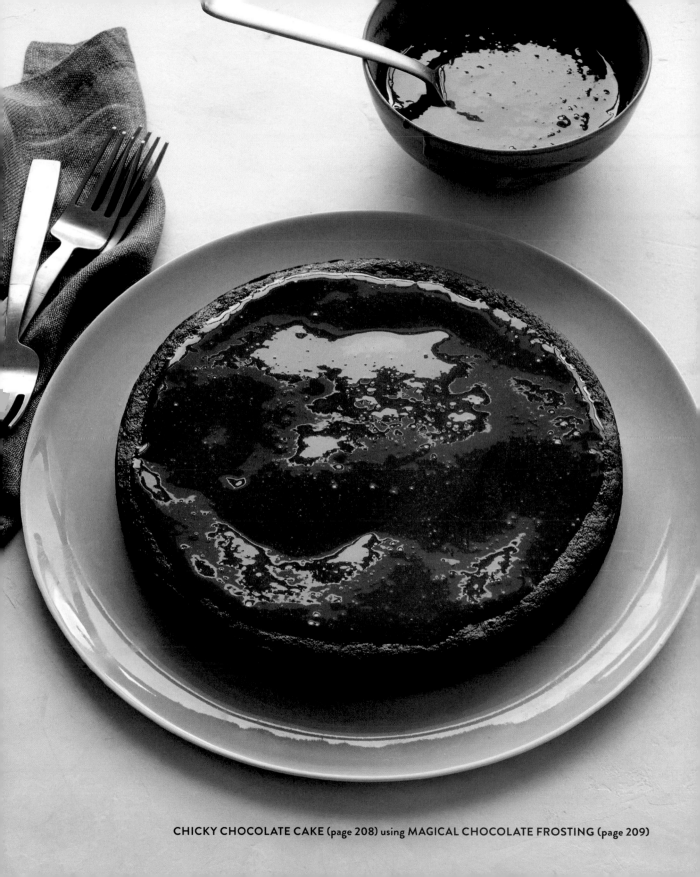

CHICKY CHOCOLATE CAKE (page 208) using MAGICAL CHOCOLATE FROSTING (page 209)

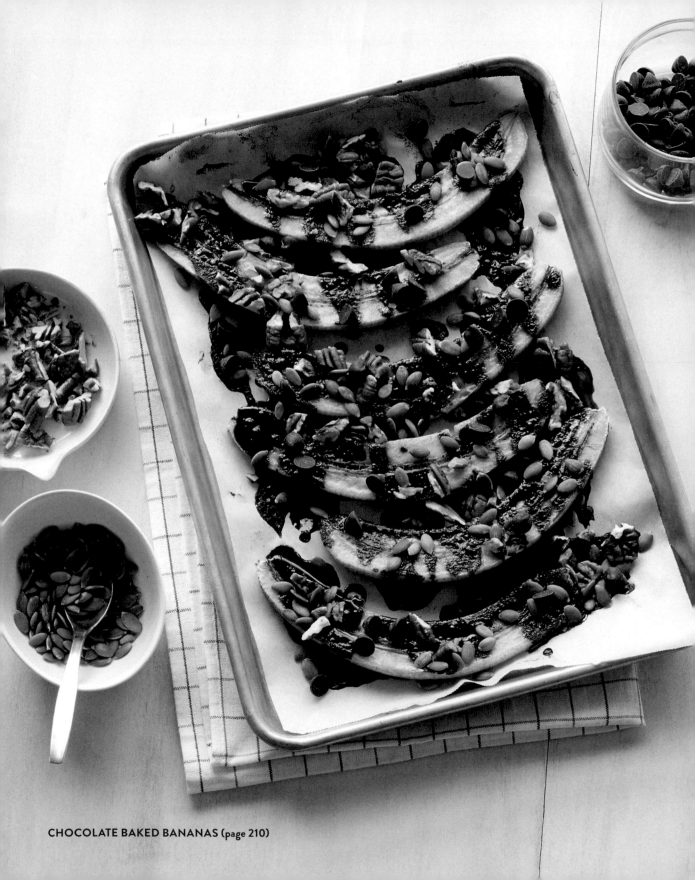

CHOCOLATE BAKED BANANAS (page 210)

LENTIL BOLOGNESE

MAKES 4 SERVINGS

Impress guests—and yourself!—with this pasta dish. The red wine adds flavor as the alcohol burns off, and the almond meal adds wonderful texture and that "extra something." Don't skip it!

⅓ cup red wine

1 cup diced onion

½ cup minced carrot

1 tablespoon dried oregano leaves

1 teaspoon vegan Worcestershire sauce

¾ teaspoon smoked paprika

½ teaspoon sea salt

¼ teaspoon ground nutmeg

1½ cups cooked brown or green lentils

¼ cup chopped sun-dried tomatoes

1 can (28 ounces) diced tomatoes (use fire-roasted, if you'd like a spicy kick)

2–3 tablespoons minced dates

1 pound dry pasta

½ cup almond meal (toast until lightly golden if you want extra flavor)

In a large pot over high heat, combine the wine, onion, carrot, oregano, Worcestershire sauce, paprika, salt, and nutmeg. Cook for 5 minutes, stirring frequently. Add the lentils, sun-dried tomatoes, diced tomatoes, and dates, and bring to a boil. Reduce the heat to low, cover, and cook for 20 to 25 minutes.

While the sauce is simmering, prepare the pasta according to package directions. Once the pasta is almost cooked (still having some "bite," not mushy), drain and return it to the cooking pot.

Add the almond meal to the sauce, stir to incorporate, and cook for a couple of minutes. Taste, season as desired, and toss with the pasta before serving.

IDEA: Instead of pasta, try serving with cooked polenta or a cooked whole grain.

NUTRITIONAL FACTS
Per serving: 754 calories, 31 g protein, 132 g carbohydrates, 14 g sugar, 11 g total fat, 12% calories from fat, 17 g fiber, 622 mg sodium

ITALIAN BEAN BURGERS

MAKES 9 BURGERS

Truly delicious. The seasonings in these burgers combine for a special flavor. They will become your new favorite!

- 2 cans (14 or 15 ounces each) chickpeas, drained and rinsed
- 1 medium–large clove garlic, cut in half
- 2 tablespoons tomato paste
- 1½ tablespoons red wine vinegar (can substitute apple cider vinegar)
- 1 tablespoon tahini
- 1 teaspoon Dijon mustard
- ½ teaspoon onion powder

- Scant ½ teaspoon sea salt
- 2 tablespoons chopped fresh oregano
- ⅓ cup roughly chopped fresh basil leaves
- 1 cup rolled oats
- ⅓ cup chopped sun-dried tomatoes (not packed in oil)
- ½ cup roughly chopped kalamata or green olives

In a food processor, combine the chickpeas, garlic, tomato paste, vinegar, tahini, mustard, onion powder, and salt. Puree until fully combined. Add the oregano, basil, and oats, and pulse briefly. (You want to combine the ingredients but retain some of the basil's texture.) Finally, pulse in the sun-dried tomatoes and olives, again maintaining some texture. Transfer the mixture to a bowl and refrigerate, covered, for 30 minutes or longer.

Preheat the oven to 400°F. Line a baking sheet with parchment paper.

Use an ice cream scoop to scoop the mixture onto the prepared baking sheet, flattening to shape into patties. Bake for about 20 minutes, flipping the burgers halfway through. Alternatively, you can cook the burgers in a non-stick skillet over medium heat for 6 to 8 minutes per side, or until golden brown. Serve.

SERVING IDEAS: Serve on whole grain burger buns with fixings, in whole grain pitas, or on top of a salad.

IDEA: Try making these as "meatballs," instead. Use a small cookie scoop and place the "meatballs" on a parchment-lined baking sheet. Bake at 400°F for 16 to 17 minutes, or until they are firm. (Don't overbake, or they will dry out.)

NUTRITIONAL FACTS
Per burger: 148 calories, 6 g protein, 23 g carbohydrates, 4 g sugar, 4 g total fat, 23% calories from fat, 6 g fiber, 387 mg sodium

EDAMAME-AVO PASTA

MAKES 4 SERVINGS

This sauce can be prepared in minutes and is lusciously satisfying! This is a very kid-friendly pasta, as well.

½ cup edamame, blanched (see Edamame Note)

1 cup cubed or sliced avocado (1½–2 small or medium avocados)

¼ cup parsley leaves (see Parsley Note)

1 small–medium clove garlic

½ tablespoon chickpea miso

1 teaspoon pure maple syrup

2–2½ tablespoons lemon juice

¾–1 teaspoon sea salt

1¼–1½ cups water

1 pound dry pasta

3 tablespoons sliced kalamata olives for serving (optional)

In a blender, combine the edamame, avocado, parsley, garlic, miso, syrup, 2 tablespoons of the lemon juice, ¾ teaspoon of the salt, and 1¼ cups of the water. Puree until very smooth. If it's very thick and not pureeing, add the remaining ¼ cup water. Taste, and add the remaining ¼ teaspoon salt and ½ tablespoon lemon juice, if desired. (Note that if you are adding olives to your final pasta dish, they will also add saltiness.)

When ready to serve, cook the pasta according to package directions. Drain and return the pasta to the pot (not over heat). Add the pasta sauce and toss thoroughly, adding the olives (if using). Serve immediately!

EDAMAME NOTE • Add the edamame to a pot of boiling water. Cook for 4 to 5 minutes, then rinse in a colander under very cold water. If you cannot consume soy, try substituting green chickpeas.

PARSLEY NOTE • Parsley really brightens the color of this puree. If you aren't fond of the flavor, you can substitute fresh basil leaves or omit it altogether.

SERVING NOTE • This sauce will oxidize slightly, so is best served the same day you've prepared it, optimally within a few hours.

NUTRITIONAL FACTS
Per serving: 599 calories, 22 g protein, 104 g carbohydrates, 4 g sugar, 10 g total fat, 14% calories from fat, 9 g fiber, 535 mg sodium

10-MINUTE STIR-FRY

MAKES 3 SERVINGS

Prepare the rice in advance, and you will have this stir-fry ready in about 10 minutes!

1 cup diced bell peppers or carrots

1 cup corn kernels or green peas (or a combination of both)

½ cup sliced green onions or chives (if using chives, add at the end of cooking)

⅓ cup diced celery

5 cups precooked brown rice or quinoa

1 cup diced precooked potatoes (or ½ cup more rice)

¼–⅓ cup tamari

1–2 tablespoons water

Sea salt to taste (optional)

Freshly ground black pepper to taste (optional)

In a large nonstick skillet over high or medium-high heat, combine the bell peppers or carrots, corn or green peas, green onions, and celery, stirring occasionally. Cook for 3 to 4 minutes, then add the rice, potatoes (if using), and ¼ cup of the tamari. Cook for another 3 to 4 minutes, stirring a couple of times. Add the water if the mixture is sticking. Heat the rice through, and toast it a little in spots, if desired. If using chives, add those and stir. Taste, add the remaining tamari, and season with salt and black pepper, if desired. Serve.

Shown in color insert pages

NUTRITIONAL FACTS

Per serving: 532 calories, 14 g protein, 112 g carbohydrates, 5 g sugar, 4 g total fat, 6% calories from fat, 9 g fiber, 1,372 mg sodium

LENTIL MUSHROOM TACO MIX

MAKES 4 SERVINGS

This mixture can be heated on the stovetop or popped into the oven. Pair it with brown rice, taco shells, or whole grain tortillas and fixings, and you're all set.

3 cups cooked brown lentils (see Lentil Note)

¾–1 pound minced mushrooms (2½–3 cups)

½ cup minced bell pepper (any color)

1 tablespoon dried oregano

1 tablespoon ground cumin

2 teaspoons chili powder

1½ teaspoons onion powder

1 teaspoon garlic powder

1 teaspoon chipotle hot sauce

1 teaspoon vegan Worcestershire sauce

¼ teaspoon allspice

¼ teaspoon crushed red-pepper flakes (or fresh minced hot pepper to taste; see Hot Pepper Note)

¾–1 teaspoon sea salt

2–2½ tablespoons lime juice

In a large bowl, combine the lentils, mushrooms, bell pepper, oregano, cumin, chili powder, onion powder, garlic powder, hot sauce, Worcestershire sauce, allspice, red-pepper flakes, and ¾ teaspoon of the salt.

Heat a nonstick skillet over medium-high heat. Add the mixture and cook, stirring occasionally, for about 10 minutes. If the mixture sticks during cooking (the mushrooms will release some moisture), add a teaspoon or two of water. Add 2 tablespoons of the lime juice, and stir through. Season with more hot sauce, the remaining ¼ teaspoon salt, and the remaining ½ tablespoon lime juice, if desired, and serve!

SERVING SUGGESTIONS: Serve in taco shells, on a taco salad, on rice, or in tortillas. Top with shredded lettuce, chopped tomatoes, chopped green onions, avocado or guacamole, or any other fixings you like!

LENTIL NOTE • Precooked lentils help bring this mix together quickly. Whenever you have time to cook brown lentils, make extra and store enough for this recipe in the fridge (for up to 5 days) or freezer (for months).

HOT PEPPER NOTE • If you'd prefer chopped jalapeño or another hot pepper, add to your taste.

NUTRITIONAL FACTS
Per serving: 213 calories, 16 g protein, 38 g carbohydrates, 3 g sugar, 1 g total fat, 6% calories from fat, 11 g fiber, 501 mg sodium

TEX-MEX RICE 'N' BEANS

MAKES 4 SERVINGS

This dish is outstanding on its own, or add a dollop of Green-with-Envy Guacamole (page 67).

1½ cups chopped bell pepper

1–1½ cups chopped onion

1 tablespoon dried oregano

2 teaspoons chili powder

½ tablespoon paprika

½ tablespoon ground cumin

1 teaspoon garlic powder

½ teaspoon cinnamon

Rounded ½ teaspoon sea salt

2 tablespoons water + 2½ cups water (boiled, if using an instant pot)

½ cup dried red lentils

1 cup uncooked brown rice (can substitute quinoa; see Note)

2 cans (15 ounces each) black beans, rinsed and drained

¼ cup tomato paste

1 bay leaf

2 tablespoons lime juice

Hot sauce to taste (optional)

In an instant pot, combine the bell pepper, onion, oregano, chili powder, paprika, cumin, garlic powder, cinnamon, salt, and 2 tablespoons of the water, and set to the sauté function. Cook for 3 to 4 minutes, stirring frequently. Turn off the sauté function and add the lentils, rice, beans, tomato paste, bay leaf, and the remaining 2½ cups water. Stir, cover the instant pot, and set to high pressure for 20 minutes. After 20 minutes, you can manually release the pressure or let it naturally release. Stir in the lime juice, taste, and season as desired. Add the hot sauce (if using), and serve.

STOVETOP VARIATION: In a large pot over high heat, combine the bell pepper, onion, oregano, chili powder, paprika, cumin, garlic powder, cinnamon, salt, and 2 tablespoons of the water. Sauté for 4 to 5 minutes, stirring frequently. Add the lentils, rice, beans, tomato paste, bay leaf, and the remaining 2½ cups water. Bring to a boil over high heat, reduce the heat to low, cover the pot, and cook for 35 minutes, or until the rice is tender. Stir in the lime juice, taste, and season as desired. Add the hot sauce (if using), and serve.

NOTE • You can use quinoa instead of rice, and the cooking time will be reduced if you do. In an instant pot, cook for about 10 minutes, and on the stovetop, cook for about 20 minutes.

Shown in color insert pages

NUTRITIONAL FACTS
Per serving: 525 calories, 24 g protein, 103 g carbohydrates, 7 g sugar, 3 g total fat, 5% calories from fat, 25 g fiber, 898 mg sodium

GREEN CHICKPEA FALAFEL

MAKES 4 SERVINGS

Green chickpeas bring a fresh dimension to falafel. You will find them in the frozen vegetables section of your grocery store.

1 bag (14 ounces) green chickpeas, thawed (about 3½ cups; see Note)

½ cup fresh flat-leaf parsley leaves

½ cup fresh cilantro leaves

1½ tablespoons freshly squeezed lemon juice

2 medium-large cloves garlic

2 teaspoons ground cumin

½ teaspoon turmeric

1 teaspoon ground coriander

1 teaspoon sea salt

¼–½ teaspoon crushed red-pepper flakes

1 cup rolled oats

In a food processor, combine the chickpeas, parsley, cilantro, lemon juice, garlic, cumin, turmeric, coriander, salt, and red-pepper flakes. (Use ¼ teaspoon if you like it mild and ½ teaspoon if you like it spicier.) Process until the mixture breaks down and begins to smooth out. Add the oats and pulse a few times to work them in. Refrigerate for 30 minutes, if possible.

Preheat the oven to 400°F. Line a baking sheet with parchment paper.

Use a cookie scoop to take small scoops of the mixture, 1 to 1½ tablespoons each. Place falafel balls on the prepared baking sheet. Bake for 11 to 12 minutes, until the falafel balls begin to firm (they will still be tender inside) and turn golden in spots.

SERVING IDEA: Serve with whole grain pitas, lettuce, chopped cucumber, and chopped tomato. Drizzle with Lightened Tahini Sauce (page 82).

NOTE • If you don't have enough of the green chickpeas, you can substitute a combination of half cooked chickpeas, half frozen green peas.

Shown in color insert pages

NUTRITIONAL FACTS
Per serving: 253 calories, 12 g protein, 43 g carbohydrates, 5 g sugar, 4 g total fat, 14% calories from fat, 10 g fiber, 601 mg sodium

RAD THAI!

MAKES 4 SERVINGS

This dish has all the flavor of a traditional pad thai and is deliciously low in fat.

⅓ cup water

1 tablespoon almond or peanut butter

¼ cup lime juice

3 tablespoons tamari

3 tablespoons ketchup

3 tablespoons coconut nectar or pure maple syrup

1 tablespoon peeled, roughly chopped ginger

2 cloves garlic, sliced or chopped

¼ teaspoon sea salt

¼ teaspoon red-pepper flakes

8 ounces dry rice noodles, such as stick or vermicelli noodles

1 cup thinly sliced red pepper

1 cup matchstick-cut carrots

½ cup sliced green onion

1 cup mung bean sprouts

¼ cup chopped cilantro

1 tablespoon chopped peanuts (optional)

4 lime wedges

Soft-Baked Tamari Tofu (optional; page 175)

In a blender, combine the water, nut butter, lime juice, tamari, ketchup, nectar or syrup, ginger, garlic, salt, and red-pepper flakes. Puree until smooth. Set aside. Cook the noodles according to package directions. Once just tender (do not overcook or they will become mushy), drain. Add the sauce to the cooking pot and place over low heat. Add the cooked noodles, red pepper, carrots, and green onion. Mix until the noodles are coated evenly with the sauce. Once warmed through, add the sprouts and cilantro. Top with the peanuts (if using), and serve immediately with the lime wedges. Serve each portion with some Soft-Baked Tamari Tofu (if using) broken up into each bowl.

Shown in color insert pages

NUTRITIONAL FACTS
Per serving: 324 calories, 7 g protein, 69 g carbohydrates, 15 g sugar, 3 g total fat, 7% calories from fat, 4 g fiber, 1,059 mg sodium

SIDES

LEMONY ROASTED CAULIFLOWER

MAKES 3 SERVINGS

Roasted cauliflower gets a puckery pop with lemon juice and a background note of smoked paprika.

3–4 tablespoons lemon juice
½ tablespoon tahini
¼ teaspoon smoked paprika

4½–5 cups cauliflower florets (about 1 medium to large head)
¼ teaspoon sea salt
Freshly ground black pepper to taste (optional)

Preheat the oven to 450°F. Line a baking sheet with parchment paper.

In a large bowl, whisk together the lemon juice, tahini, and smoked paprika. Add the cauliflower and toss to coat. Transfer the cauliflower to the prepared baking sheet, scraping all of the lemon sauce over the cauliflower. Sprinkle with the salt. Bake for 25 to 30 minutes, stirring a couple of times, until golden. (Larger pieces will take longer to cook.) Remove, season with salt and pepper (if using) to taste, and serve.

Shown in color insert pages

NUTRITIONAL FACTS

Per serving: 51 calories, 3 g protein, 7 g carbohydrates, 3 g sugar, 2 g total fat, 33% calories from fat, 4 g fiber, 368 mg sodium

SOFT-BAKED TAMARI TOFU

MAKES 4 SERVINGS

This is the simplest tofu dish, yet it's so ridiculously tasty! Serve it over rice, quinoa, greens, or noodles, or with Rad Thai! (page 171) or Thai Corn and Sweet Potato Stew (page 115).

3 tablespoons tamari

1 package (16 ounces) medium-firm tofu

Preheat the oven to 425°F. In an ovenproof dish just large enough to hold the tofu, add about half of the tamari. Use several paper towels to pat or squeeze some of the excess moisture from the tofu. Add the tofu to the dish, breaking it up slightly. Sprinkle the remaining tamari over the tofu. Bake for 20 to 25 minutes, or until the tofu is browned and drying in spots. Serve, spooning out tofu with some of the remaining tamari.

NUTRITIONAL FACTS

Per serving: 87 calories, 10 g protein, 3 g carbohydrates, 1 g sugar, 5 g total fat, 46% calories from fat, 1 g fiber, 768 mg sodium

BROILED ASPARAGUS

MAKES 3 SERVINGS

Asparagus is at its best when you keep it simple. Just a little seasoning and broiling does the trick!

1 pound asparagus	¼ teaspoon sea salt
1 teaspoon lemon juice	Lemon pepper (optional)

Set the oven or toaster oven to broil. Line a baking sheet with parchment paper.

Wash and trim the asparagus. (Use a knife or break off ends where they naturally snap.) Pat the asparagus dry, and transfer to the prepared baking sheet. Sprinkle with the lemon juice, toss to coat, and then sprinkle with the salt. Broil for 5 to 6 minutes, or until the asparagus turns bright green. Remove, sprinkle with the lemon pepper (if using), and serve.

Shown in color insert pages

NUTRITIONAL FACTS
Per serving: 17 calories, 2 g protein, 3 g carbohydrates, 1 g sugar, 0.2 g total fat, 8% calories from fat, 2 g fiber, 206 mg sodium

SESAME BROCCOLI

MAKES 3 SERVINGS

Steamed broccoli is tossed in a tahini-based sauce then topped off with sesame seeds. A simple, tasty side dish!

1	tablespoon tahini	1	teaspoon freshly grated ginger
1½	tablespoons coconut nectar	¼	teaspoon garlic powder
1½	tablespoons tamari	4–5	cups broccoli florets
1	teaspoon apple cider vinegar	2	teaspoons sesame seeds (raw or lightly toasted)

In a large bowl, whisk together the tahini, nectar, tamari, vinegar, ginger, and garlic powder. Set aside. Place a steamer basket in a large pot with 2" of water. Bring to a boil over high heat. Place the broccoli in the basket and steam for 3 to 4 minutes, or until it turns bright green and is just becoming tender. Drain and pat dry the broccoli. Add the broccoli to the marinade, and toss to coat thoroughly. Sprinkle with the sesame seeds and serve.

Shown in color insert pages

NUTRITIONAL FACTS
Per serving: 115 calories, 5 g protein, 17 g carbohydrates, 8 g sugar, 4 g total fat, 33% calories from fat, 5 g fiber, 558 mg sodium

MOREISH LEMONY QUINOA

MAKES 3 SERVINGS

Combined with lemon, tahini, and seasonings in this easy recipe, this quinoa is delectable.

1 cup dry quinoa, rinsed and drained	2 tablespoons tahini
1¾ cups water	3–4 tablespoons fresh lemon juice
2½ tablespoons tamari	½ teaspoon garlic powder

In a large saucepan over high heat, combine the quinoa and water. Bring to a boil, stir, then reduce the heat to low. Cover and cook for 11 minutes. In a small bowl, combine the tamari, tahini, lemon juice, and garlic powder. Whisk to combine. Once the quinoa is cooked, turn off the heat and stir in the tahini mixture. Cover again, let sit for a couple of minutes, and serve.

NUTRITIONAL FACTS
Per serving: 281 calories, 11 g protein, 40 g carbohydrates, 4 g sugar, 9 g total fat, 27% calories from fat, 5 g fiber, 861 mg sodium

MINUTE GARLIC BREAD

MAKES 4 SERVINGS

With this simple technique, you will have delicious garlic bread in minutes.

1 loaf whole grain sliced baguette or other sliced whole grain bread, frozen

1–2 large cloves garlic

Few pinches of sea salt

2–3 teaspoons nutritional yeast or 1–2 tablespoons Balsamic Drizzle (page 83; optional)

Preheat the oven to 400°F. Line a baking sheet with parchment paper.

Separate the slices of bread while still frozen, and rub the garlic on one side of each slice of bread. (The garlic will be worn down and "grated" by the frozen bread.) Sprinkle with the salt and place on the prepared baking sheet. Bake for 8 to 9 minutes, or until lightly browned and fragrant. Serve, sprinkling with the yeast or the Balsamic Drizzle (if using).

NUTRITIONAL FACTS

Per serving: 105 calories, 4 g protein, 20 g carbohydrates, 2 g sugar, 1 g total fat, 8% calories from fat, 1 g fiber, 448 mg sodium

MARINATED GREEN BEANS

MAKES 3 SERVINGS

These beans are fresh and vibrant, and if you have leftovers, they'll develop a lovely pickled flavor.

½–¾ pound green beans, ends trimmed
1 tablespoon nutritional yeast
1 teaspoon Dijon mustard
1 tablespoon apple cider vinegar

2 teaspoons coconut nectar or pure maple syrup
Rounded ¼ teaspoon sea salt
Freshly ground black pepper to taste (optional)

Place a large pot of water over high heat, and bring to a boil. Add the green beans and cook for 2 to 3 minutes. Run the beans under cold water to stop the cooking process. Drain the beans and pat dry, if needed. In a large bowl, combine the yeast, mustard, vinegar, nectar or syrup, salt, and pepper (if using). Whisk until thoroughly combined. Add the green beans, and toss to coat thoroughly. Let sit for 30 minutes, then serve.

Shown in color insert pages

NUTRITIONAL FACTS
Per serving: 47 calories, 3 g protein, 9 g carbohydrates, 4 g sugar, 0.4 g total fat, 8% calories from fat, 3 g fiber, 335 mg sodium

MUSHROOM "BACON" TOPPER

MAKES 4 SERVINGS (AS A TOPPING)

Thinly sliced shiitake mushrooms baked in a smoky marinade transform into a tasty "bacon" that is fabulous on pasta, salads, and more.

½ pound shiitake mushrooms, stems removed (see Note)

2½ teaspoons balsamic vinegar

2½ teaspoons tamari

1 tablespoon pure maple syrup

½ teaspoon smoked paprika

½ teaspoon Dijon mustard

¼ teaspoon liquid smoke

Freshly ground pepper or lemon pepper to taste

Preheat the oven to 400°F. Line a baking sheet with parchment paper.

Use a damp paper towel to clean the mushrooms. Slice the mushrooms thinly. In a large bowl, combine the vinegar, tamari, syrup, paprika, mustard, liquid smoke, and pepper. Whisk thoroughly. Add the mushrooms and stir to coat with the marinade. Transfer the mushrooms to the prepared baking sheet. Bake for 16 to 17 minutes, tossing once. Turn off the heat and let the mushrooms sit in the warm oven for 10 minutes, tossing once during this time. Remove and let cool. Serve on salads, soups, pizzas, and more.

NOTE • Purchase just over ½ pound of mushrooms, and then remove the woody stems, which are not edible. If you don't want to discard the stems altogether, you can save them to make a mushroom or vegetable stock.

NUTRITIONAL FACTS
Per serving: 45 calories, 2 g protein, 9 g carbohydrates, 6 g sugar, 0.4 g total fat, 7% calories from fat, 2 g fiber, 233 mg sodium

FOCACCIA

MAKES 2 SERVINGS

This focaccia is loaded with flavor, with very little fat.

¾ cup warm water

1 packet quick-rise yeast (can use standard yeast; see Yeast Note)

½ tablespoon coconut sugar or pure maple syrup

2 cups white wheat flour (see Flour Note)

Rounded ¼ teaspoon sea salt

1½–2 teaspoons chopped fresh rosemary leaves (can substitute thyme)

Scant ½ teaspoon coarse salt

Freshly ground black pepper (to taste) or lemon pepper

In a small bowl, combine the warm water, yeast, and sugar or syrup. (The water should be warm but not hot, as hot will kill the yeast but water that is too cold will not activate it.) Whisk well, and let stand for about 5 minutes, or until foamy.

Meanwhile, in a large bowl, combine the flour and sea salt, and mix. Once the yeast mixture is foamy, add it to the flour. Use a large spoon to work the mixture together. Once the dough comes together, either knead the dough inside the bowl or lightly flour the countertop and transfer the dough there for kneading. Knead for just a couple of minutes. Lightly coat the inside of a large bowl with cooking spray and transfer the dough to that bowl. Cover with plastic wrap. Place the bowl on a countertop in a warm but not hot area to rest and rise for 30 minutes or more.

Preheat the oven to 450°F for at least a half-hour. Lightly coat a large piece of parchment with cooking spray.

Transfer the dough to the prepared parchment, and begin to press it into shape with your fingers. Focaccia can be round, or squarish, or whatever shape you like. Use your fingers to poke into the surface of the dough, leaving small indentations all over. Sprinkle on the rosemary, coarse salt, and pepper. Bake for 12 to 15 minutes, or until golden on the edges. Remove, let cool slightly, and cut to serve.

YEAST NOTE • You can use a standard baking yeast, if you prefer. If you do, give the dough at least 1½ hours to rise.

FLOUR NOTE • You can also substitute whole wheat pastry flour for this crust. The white wheat flour gives a softer, lighter texture, however.

NUTRITIONAL FACTS
Per serving: 434 calories, 17 g protein, 91 g carbohydrates, 4 g sugar, 3 g total fat, 6% calories from fat, 14 g fiber, 973 mg sodium

COCONUT CURRY RICE

MAKES 3 SERVINGS

This rice boasts a beautiful bright yellow color and has a delicate curried, creamy flavor. It's easy to make and looks and tastes so impressive!

1   cup uncooked brown rice or brown basmati rice

1⅓ cups water

1   small can (5.5 ounces) light coconut milk

2   tablespoons freshly squeezed lime juice

1   teaspoon mild curry powder
    Rounded ¼ teaspoon sea salt

¼   teaspoon turmeric powder

3–4 tablespoons chopped cilantro for serving (optional)
    Lime wedges for serving

In a saucepan, combine the rice, water, coconut milk, lime juice, curry powder, salt, and turmeric. Bring to a boil over high heat, stir, then reduce the heat to low. Cover and cook for 35 to 45 minutes, until the liquid is absorbed and the rice is tender. Turn off the heat and let the rice sit, covered, for 5 minutes. Stir in the cilantro (if using), and serve with the lime wedges.

Shown in color insert pages

NUTRITIONAL FACTS
Per serving: 298 calories, 6 g protein, 56 g carbohydrates, 2 g sugar, 6 g total fat, 17% calories from fat, 4 g fiber, 303 mg sodium

TERIYAKI CHICKPEAS

MAKES 7 SERVINGS

Chickpeas and teriyaki pair beautifully and will have you coming back for more.

2 cans (15 ounces each) chickpeas, rinsed and drained

1½ tablespoons tamari

1 tablespoon pure maple syrup

1 tablespoon lemon juice

½–¾ teaspoon garlic powder

½ teaspoon ground ginger

½ teaspoon blackstrap molasses

Preheat the oven to 450°F. Line a baking sheet with parchment paper.

In a large mixing bowl, combine the chickpeas, tamari, syrup, lemon juice, garlic powder, ginger, and molasses. Toss to combine. Spread evenly on the prepared baking sheet and bake for 20 to 25 minutes, or until the marinade is absorbed. Serve warm, or refrigerate to enjoy later.

IDEA: Beyond snacking, these chickpeas make a delicious and satisfying topper for salads, pasta dishes, soups, and stir-fries.

NUTRITIONAL FACTS
Per serving: 120 calories, 6 g protein, 20 g carbohydrates, 5 g sugar, 2 g total fat, 15% calories from fat, 5 g fiber, 382 mg sodium

SAVORY SWEET POTATO FRIES

MAKES 4 SERVINGS

The savory seasonings offer delectable flavor contrast to the natural sweetness of the sweet potatoes. These fries are keepers!

1½ tablespoons balsamic vinegar

½ tablespoon coconut nectar

1 teaspoon dried oregano leaves

½ teaspoon dried rosemary

½ teaspoon dried basil

½ tablespoon Dijon mustard

½ teaspoon sea salt

3 pounds orange-fleshed sweet potatoes (look for garnet or jewel yams), washed and cut into wedges

Preheat the oven to 425°F. Line a large, rimmed baking sheet with parchment paper, and lightly coat the surface of the parchment with cooking spray.

In a large bowl, whisk together the vinegar, nectar, oregano, rosemary, basil, mustard, and salt. Add the potato wedges to the mixture and toss to coat. Place on the prepared baking sheet, and pour any remaining liquid over the wedges. Bake, flipping the wedges once or twice, for 55 to 65 minutes or longer, or until the sweet potatoes have softened and are also caramelized (delicious!) in spots. Serve.

NUTRITIONAL FACTS
Per serving: 201 calories, 4 g protein, 46 g carbohydrates, 16 g sugar, 0.5 g total fat, 2% calories from fat, 7 g fiber, 414 mg sodium

SWEET POTATO CRISPS

MAKES 3 SERVINGS

You might want to eat the full batch of these nibbly chips straight out of the oven. If you're able to resist, try them on top of dinner salads or soups.

1 pound sweet potatoes
½ tablespoon balsamic vinegar

½ tablespoon pure maple syrup
Rounded ¼ teaspoon sea salt

Preheat the oven to 400°F. Line a large baking sheet with parchment paper.

Peel the sweet potatoes, then use the peeler to continue to make sweet potato peelings. (Alternatively, you can push peeled sweet potatoes through a food processor slicing blade.) Transfer the peelings to a large mixing bowl and use your hands to toss with the vinegar and syrup, coating them as evenly as possible. Spread the peelings on the prepared baking sheet, spacing well. Sprinkle with the salt. Bake for 30 minutes, tossing once or twice. The pieces around the edges of the pan can get brown quickly, so move the chips around during baking. Turn off the oven and let the chips sit in the residual heat for 20 minutes, stir again, and let sit for another 15 to 20 minutes, until they crisp up. Remove, and snack!

Shown in color insert pages

NUTRITIONAL FACTS
Per serving: 94 calories, 2 g protein, 22 g carbohydrates, 8 g sugar, 0.1 g total fat, 1% calories from fat, 3 g fiber, 326 mg sodium

MOROCCAN-ROASTED CHICKPEAS

MAKES 3 SERVINGS

Warm, earthy spices coat the chickpeas, and roasting enhances the flavors. Delicious!

1 can (15 ounces) chickpeas, rinsed and drained

1 tablespoon apple cider vinegar

½ teaspoon smoked paprika

½ teaspoon ground cumin

½ teaspoon cinnamon

½ teaspoon dried basil leaves

½ teaspoon pure maple syrup

¼ teaspoon sea salt

Preheat the oven to 425°F. Line a baking sheet with parchment paper.

In a large mixing bowl, combine the chickpeas, vinegar, paprika, cumin, cinnamon, basil, syrup, and salt. Toss to combine. Spread evenly on the prepared baking sheet and bake for 15 to 20 minutes, or until the marinade is absorbed. Serve warm, or refrigerate to enjoy later.

Shown in color insert pages

NUTRITIONAL FACTS
Per serving: 134 calories, 7 g protein, 22 g carbohydrates, 4 g sugar, 3 g total fat, 17% calories from fat, 6 g fiber, 389 mg sodium

CHEESY CAULI BAKE
MAKES 6 SERVINGS

This cauliflower is so irresistible in its creamy, tangy sauce that you might find yourself eating it as a main dish with quinoa or greens 'n' beans. A double-batch might be in order!

3 tablespoons tahini

2 tablespoons nutritional yeast

1 tablespoon lemon juice

½ teaspoon pure maple syrup or agave nectar

½ teaspoon sea salt

½ cup + 1 tablespoon plain nondairy milk

3–3½ cups cauliflower florets, cut or broken in small pieces

Topping

1 tablespoon almond meal or breadcrumbs

½ tablespoon nutritional yeast

Pinch sea salt

Preheat the oven to 425°F. Use cooking spray to lightly coat the bottom and sides of an 8" x 8" (or similar size) baking dish.

In a small bowl, whisk together the tahini, nutritional yeast, lemon juice, maple syrup or agave nectar, and salt. Gradually whisk in the milk until it all comes together smoothly. In the baking dish, add the cauliflower and pour in the sauce, stir thoroughly to coat the cauliflower. Cover with foil and bake for 25 to 30 minutes, stirring only once, until the cauliflower is tender.

In a small bowl, toss together the topping ingredients. Remove the foil from the cauliflower, and sprinkle on the topping. Return to the oven and set oven to broil. Allow to cook for a minute or so until the topping is golden brown. Remove, let sit for a few minutes, then serve.

NOTE • If the sauce separates a little after baking, just stir through as much as you can, then let bake again uncovered for a few minutes, and then to broil with the topping.

Shown in color insert pages

NUTRITIONAL FACTS
Per serving: 87 calories, 5 g protein, 7 g carbohydrate, 2 g sugar, 5 g total fat, 50% calories from fat, 3 g fiber, 270 mg sodium

DESSERTS

NO-BAKE BROWNIE BITES

MAKES ABOUT 23

These chocolaty treats are like little brownie bites, and so easy to make.

1½ cups pitted dates

½ cup raisins

1 cup rolled oats

2 tablespoons pumpkin seeds

¼ cup cocoa powder

2 tablespoons chocolate plant-based protein powder (optional)

⅛ teaspoon sea salt

1 teaspoon pure vanilla extract

3 tablespoons sugar-free, nondairy chocolate chips (optional)

In a food processor, combine the dates, raisins, oats, and pumpkin seeds. Process until the mixture is crumbly. Add the cocoa, protein powder (if using), salt, and vanilla. Process again, and let the processor run until the mixture begins to get sticky and form clumps. At this point, add the chocolate chips (if using), and pulse until a ball forms on the blade. Remove the bowl, and roll small scoops (about 1 tablespoon each) of the mixture into balls. Continue until all of the mixture is used. Transfer to an airtight container in the fridge, where they will keep for a couple of weeks, or to the freezer, where they will keep for a couple of months.

NUTRITIONAL FACTS

Per 3-ball serving: 168 calories, 4 g protein, 38 g carbohydrates, 24 g sugar, 2 g total fat, 11% calories from fat, 5 g fiber, 41 mg sodium

BLENDER BANANA SNACK CAKE

MAKES 9 SERVINGS

Baking doesn't get much easier than this. Everything goes into the blender, then into the oven. Presto, banana cake!

¼ cup coconut nectar or pure maple syrup

¼ cup water

2 teaspoons vanilla

1 teaspoon cinnamon

½ teaspoon nutmeg

¼ teaspoon sea salt

3½ cups sliced, well-ripened bananas

1 cup whole grain spelt flour

½ cup rolled oats

2 teaspoons baking powder

Preheat the oven to 350°F. Lightly coat an 8" x 8" pan with cooking spray and line the bottom of the pan with parchment paper.

In a blender, combine the nectar or syrup, water, vanilla, cinnamon, nutmeg, salt, and 3 cups of the sliced bananas. Puree until smooth. Add the flour, oats, baking powder, and the remaining ½ cup of bananas. Pulse a couple of times, until just combined. (Don't puree; you don't want to overwork the flour.) Transfer the mixture into the baking dish, using a spatula to scrape down the sides of the bowl. Bake for 30 to 32 minutes, until fully set. (Insert a toothpick in the center and see if it comes out clean.) Transfer the cake pan to a cooling rack. Let cool completely before cutting.

NUTRITIONAL FACTS
Per serving: 141 calories, 3 g protein, 32 g carbohydrates, 14 g sugar, 1 g total fat, 5% calories from fat, 4 g fiber, 177 mg sodium

ORANGE-MANGO CREAM

MAKES 6 SERVINGS (ABOUT 1½ CUPS)

This sauce works equally well with pancakes or French toast, or to dollop on oatmeal!

1 cup frozen mango

¼ cup soaked cashews

½ cup + 1–3 tablespoons orange juice

1–2 tablespoons coconut nectar (optional)

Pinch of sea salt

In a blender, combine the mango, cashews, and ½ cup of the juice. Puree until smooth. If the mixture is too thick to blend, add the additional 1 to 3 tablespoons of orange juice as needed. Puree again. Taste, and add the coconut nectar, if desired. Serve with fruit, Easy-as-Pie Baked Apples (page 198), or Breakfast Polenta Cakes (page 34).

NUTRITIONAL FACTS

Per serving: 56 calories, 1 g protein, 8 g carbohydrates, 6 g sugar, 2 g total fat, 37% calories from fat, 1 g fiber, 50 mg sodium

DREAMY CHOCOLATE GELATO

MAKES 3 SERVINGS (2¾ CUPS)

Dessert dreams do come true! This dreamy chocolate gelato is made with simple, healthful ingredients. No ice cream maker required!

½ cup cubed ripe avocado

2 tablespoons raw cashew or raw almond butter

½ cup low-fat nondairy milk

1 cup (packed) pitted dates

1 cup frozen, overripe, sliced bananas

¼ cup cocoa powder

½ teaspoon pure vanilla extract

⅛ teaspoon sea salt

In a high-speed blender, combine the avocado, nut butter, milk, dates, bananas, cocoa, vanilla, and salt. (If you're using a standard blender, soak the dates in warm water for about ½ hour, then drain before blending.) Puree until very smooth. Transfer to a container to freeze. The gelato will take 4 to 6 hours to completely set, but it can also be enjoyed softer set. It's up to you!

IDEA: This mixture is equally delicious served straight up as a pudding or mousse. Try serving it with fresh berries or other fruit.

NUTRITIONAL FACTS
Per serving: 320 calories, 6 g protein, 60 g carbohydrates, 39 g sugar, 11 g total fat, 28% calories from fat, 10 g fiber, 119 mg sodium

STRAWBERRY CHIA PUDDING

MAKES 2 SERVINGS

This pudding can be made at any time of year using frozen berries—and very quickly, too. The chia seeds are pureed with the berries for a creamy, smooth texture.

1½ cups frozen whole strawberries (see Strawberries Note)

3 tablespoons white chia seeds (see Chia Seeds Note)

1 tablespoon coconut nectar or pure maple syrup

1 teaspoon lemon juice
Pinch of sea salt

½ cup + 2–3 tablespoons plain low-fat nondairy milk

In a blender, combine the strawberries, chia seeds, nectar or syrup, lemon juice, salt, and ½ cup plus 2 tablespoons of the milk. Puree until the seeds are fully pulverized and the pudding begins to thicken. (It will thicken more as it cools.) Add the extra 1 tablespoon milk if needed to blend. Transfer the mixture to a large bowl or dish and refrigerate until chilled, about an hour or more. (It will thicken more with chilling, but really can be eaten right away.)

STRAWBERRIES NOTE • Frozen strawberries can be tricky to measure, since some are very large, and we don't slice or chop them before blending. Just measure the best you can. The flavor will be great whether the measure is a little generous or a little scant!

CHIA SEEDS NOTE • In this recipe, it's best to use white chia seeds, as black seeds will discolor the pudding.

Shown in color insert pages

NUTRITIONAL FACTS
Per serving: 185 calories, 4 g protein, 33 g carbohydrates, 16 g sugar, 5 g total fat, 24% calories from fat, 9 g fiber, 182 mg sodium

BANANA BREAD NICE CREAM

MAKES 3 SERVINGS (1¾ CUPS)

Here is the taste of freshly baked banana bread in a creamy, dreamy "ice cream."

½ cup (packed) pitted dates (see Note)

¼–⅓ cup plain or vanilla low-fat nondairy milk

1 tablespoon raw cashew or raw almond butter

¼ teaspoon ground nutmeg

A couple pinches of sea salt

2 cups frozen, sliced, overripe bananas

In a blender, combine the dates with ¼ cup of the milk. (If you're using a high-speed blender, that should be enough milk, but if you're using a regular blender you may need to use ⅓ cup of the milk.) Blend until smooth. Add the nut butter, nutmeg, and salt, and blend. Add about half of the bananas and puree until the mixture is smooth, then add the remaining bananas and puree again until smooth. Transfer to a container and freeze for 1 to 2 hours (for soft serve) or 4 to 5 hours or overnight for a firmer-set ice cream.

NOTE • If your dates are soft, go ahead and blend them up. If they are at all hard or chewy, soak them in boiled water for about 15 minutes. Drain off all the water before adding them to the recipe.

NUTRITIONAL FACTS
Per serving: 198 calories, 3 g protein, 44 g carbohydrates, 29 g sugar, 3 g total fat, 14% calories from fat, 5 g fiber, 205 mg sodium

EASY-AS-PIE BAKED APPLES

MAKES 4 SERVINGS

This is such a fun way to prepare baked apples! Instead of baking them whole, we cut them in half, then add toppings. They are easy to make and look impressive when served to guests.

- 4 medium apples, cored and cut in half horizontally
- 2 teaspoons lemon juice
- 16 pitted dates
- ¼ cup almond flour (or tigernut flour, for nut-free)

- 2 tablespoons coconut sugar
- 1½ teaspoons cinnamon
- ⅛ teaspoon sea salt
- ¼ cup boiled water

Preheat the oven to 400°F.

Place the apple halves, cut sides up, in a glass pie plate. Squeeze the lemon juice over the tops of the apples. Place 2 dates in the center of each apple half. In a small bowl, combine the flour, sugar, cinnamon, and salt. Mix to combine well. Distribute this filling among the centers and over the tops of the apples. Pour the water into the bottom of the pie plate. Cover with foil and bake for 30 minutes. Remove the foil after 30 minutes, and bake for another 7 to 10 minutes, to lightly brown the tops of the apples. Remove from the oven, let cool as desired, and serve.

NUTRITIONAL FACTS
Per serving: 242 calories, 3 g protein, 55 g carbohydrates, 44 g sugar, 4 g total fat, 14% calories from fat, 8 g fiber, 77 mg sodium

SALTED CARAMEL SAUCE

MAKES 4 SERVINGS (¾ CUP)

This sauce is unbelievably simple yet tastes sublime. Try it over desserts, as a dip for fruit, or even as a sauce for waffles, pancakes, or fruit parfaits.

½ cup packed dates (see Note)

⅔ cup low-fat nondairy milk

1 tablespoon almond or cashew butter (optional)

¼ teaspoon sea salt

¼ teaspoon vanilla bean powder (or ½ teaspoon pure vanilla extract)

In a blender, combine the dates, milk, nut butter, salt, and vanilla powder or extract. (This is quick and easy with a high-speed blender. With a regular blender, it will take longer.) Puree until the mixture is smooth, and also until it starts to become warm. Serve immediately or transfer to an airtight container and refrigerate for up to a week.

NOTE • If your dates aren't very soft, soak them in boiled water for 15 minutes and drain well before blending.

NUTRITIONAL FACTS
Per serving: 67 calories, 1 g protein, 16 g carbohydrates, 13 g sugar, 0.3 g total fat, 4% calories from fat, 2 g fiber, 162 mg sodium

APPLE CRISP

MAKES 4 SERVINGS

This light, healthful apple crisp is quick and easy to prepare. For a tasty variation, try substituting a portion of the apples with an equal amount of fresh pears. Try it with a small scoop of nondairy ice cream or dairy-free yogurt.

Fruit Mixture

- 3 tablespoons freshly squeezed orange juice or pressed apple juice
- 2 tablespoons coconut nectar or pure maple syrup
- 2 tablespoons water
- 1½ tablespoons freshly squeezed lemon juice
- 2 teaspoons arrowroot or tapioca powder (can substitute organic cornstarch)
- 1 teaspoon cinnamon
  Pinch of allspice

- ⅛ teaspoon sea salt
- 4–4½ cups apples, cored, cut into small chunks (peeling optional)

Crisp Topping

- 1½ tablespoons almond or cashew butter, raw or roasted
- 3 tablespoons coconut nectar or pure maple syrup
- ¾ cup rolled oats
- ½ cup oat flour
- ⅛ teaspoon sea salt

Preheat the oven to 350°F.

To make the fruit mixture: In a large bowl, combine the orange or apple juice, nectar or syrup, water, and lemon juice. Stir to combine. Add the arrowroot or tapioca powder, cinnamon, allspice, and salt, whisking thoroughly. Add the fruit and stir to coat. Transfer the mixture to an 8" x 8" (or similar size) glass baking dish.

To make the topping: In a medium bowl, combine the nut butter with the nectar or syrup, stirring until fully incorporated. Add the oats, oat flour, and salt, and mix until crumbly, using a spoon or your fingers. Sprinkle the topping evenly over the fruit. Cover with foil and bake for 35 minutes, or until the fruit is tender. Remove the foil and bake for another 10 minutes, to crisp the topping slightly. Let cool a little before serving.

Shown in color insert pages

NUTRITIONAL FACTS
Per serving: 292 calories, 6 g protein, 59 g carbohydrates, 30 g sugar, 6 g total fat, 16% calories from fat, 7 g fiber, 166 mg sodium

BANANA BREAD PUDDING

MAKES 5 SERVINGS

Call it dessert or call it breakfast. Or just call it fabulous!

6–6½ cups cubed sprouted grain bread (can use heels of bread or mix varieties)

⅓ cup pure maple syrup

2 tablespoons hemp seeds

2 tablespoons whole chia seeds

1 teaspoon cinnamon

1 teaspoon pure vanilla extract

⅛ teaspoon sea salt

1½ cups plain low-fat nondairy milk

2 cups sliced overripe bananas (about 3 small or medium)

Preheat the oven to 350°F. Lightly coat an 8" x 8" glass baking dish with cooking spray.

Place the cubed bread in the prepared dish. In a blender, combine the syrup, hemp seeds, chia seeds, cinnamon, vanilla, salt, and about half of the milk. Puree until completely smooth. Add the remaining milk and the sliced bananas. Pulse to break up the bananas. (You want them lightly mashed, not fully pureed.) Pour this mixture over the bread cubes and gently mix to combine. Bake for about 40 minutes, or until the top is golden and the bread pudding is fairly well set. (It can retain a softer, more pudding-like consistency, but it shouldn't be sloshy.) Remove from the oven and let cool slightly before serving. You can also serve it at room temperature or chilled, but warm is tastiest! (See Note.)

NOTE • If you've refrigerated leftovers, you can gently reheat them in either the same glass pan or a smaller ovenproof dish. Cover the dish with foil and bake at 350°F until the food is warmed through.

NUTRITIONAL FACTS

Per serving: 302 calories, 8 g protein, 58 g carbohydrates, 24 g sugar, 5 g total fat, 14% calories from fat, 7 g fiber, 370 mg sodium

RASPBERRY NICE CREAM

MAKES 3 SERVINGS

This easy and delightful dessert is refreshing, bright, and creamy.

2 cups frozen, sliced, overripe bananas

2 cups frozen or fresh raspberries

Pinch of sea salt

1–2 tablespoons coconut nectar or 1–1½ tablespoons pure maple syrup

In a food processor or high-speed blender (see Note), combine the bananas, raspberries, salt, and 1 tablespoon of the nectar or syrup. Puree until smooth. Taste, and add the remaining nectar or syrup, if desired. Serve immediately, if you like a soft-serve consistency, or transfer to an airtight container and freeze for an hour or more, if you like a firmer texture.

NOTE • If you don't have a high-speed blender, use a food processor, instead. A standard blender will have a hard time chugging through the frozen fruit without adding extra liquid.

NUTRITIONAL FACTS
Per serving: 193 calories, 3 g protein, 47 g carbohydrates, 24 g sugar, 1 g total fat, 6% calories from fat, 13 g fiber, 101 mg sodium

PINEAPPLE-BANANA WHIP

MAKES 3 SERVINGS (3 CUPS)

This is a twist on the popular pineapple whip that you may have seen at amusement parks. Now you can make it at home.

2 cups cubed frozen pineapple (see Pineapple Note)

1 cup sliced, frozen, overripe banana

⅓ cup + 1–2 tablespoons low-fat nondairy milk (see Milk Note)

¼ teaspoon vanilla bean powder (optional)

Small pinch of sea salt

2–3 teaspoons coconut nectar or pure maple syrup (optional)

In a food processor or high-speed blender (see Blender Note), combine the pineapple, banana, vanilla powder, salt, and ⅓ cup of the milk. Pulse to get things moving, and then puree. Add the remaining 1 to 2 tablespoons milk if needed to blend. Once the whip is smooth, taste it, and add the nectar or syrup, if desired. Serve, or transfer to an airtight container and freeze for an hour or more to set a little more firmly before serving.

PINEAPPLE NOTE • Another delicious option is to substitute frozen mango for some or all of the pineapple. Try using 1 cup of each at first, and if you love it, next time try using mango for the full 2 cups! You may want to use more maple syrup with mango.

MILK NOTE • Depending on your blender and whether you're using a room temperature banana, you may need more or less milk. Blend and add milk as needed. Just be patient, let the blender get moving, and don't overdo the milk initially.

BLENDER NOTE • If you don't have a high-speed blender, use a food processor instead. While you can use a standard blender here, it has a harder time working through the frozen fruit with this amount of liquid, so you may need more liquid than is optimal for the recipe.

NUTRITIONAL FACTS
Per serving: 109 calories, 2 g protein, 27 g carbohydrates, 18 g sugar, 0.5 g total fat, 4% calories from fat, 3 g fiber, 77 mg sodium

OATMEAL CHIPPERS

MAKES 20

Made with whole grain flours and no butter or oil, these cookies are almost too good to be true. Healthy *and* delicious!

3–3½ tablespoons almond butter (or tigernut butter, for nut-free)

¼ cup pure maple syrup

¼ cup brown rice syrup

2 teaspoons pure vanilla extract

1⅓ cups oat flour

1 cup + 2 tablespoons rolled oats

1½ teaspoons baking powder

½ teaspoon cinnamon

¼ teaspoon sea salt

2–3 tablespoons sugar-free nondairy chocolate chips

Preheat the oven to 350°F. Line a baking sheet with parchment paper.

In the bowl of a mixer, combine the almond butter, maple syrup, brown rice syrup, and vanilla. Using the paddle attachment, mix on low speed for a couple of minutes, until creamy. Turn off the mixer and add the flour, oats, baking powder, cinnamon, salt, and chocolate chips. Mix on low speed until incorporated. Place 1½-tablespoon mounds on the prepared baking sheet, spacing them 1" to 2" apart, and flatten slightly. Bake for 11 minutes, or until just set to the touch. Remove from the oven, let cool on the pan for just a minute, and then transfer the cookies to a cooling rack.

NUTRITIONAL FACTS
Per cookie: 90 calories, 2 g protein, 16 g carbohydrates, 4 g sugar, 2 g total fat, 23% calories from fat, 2 g fiber, 75 mg sodium

MANGO NICE CREAM

MAKES 4 SERVINGS

This dessert has the creamy, light texture of gelato, with the sweetness reined in. It is just delicious.

2 cups frozen mango chunks

1 cup frozen, sliced, overripe banana (can use room temperature, but must be overripe)

Pinch of sea salt

½ teaspoon pure vanilla extract

¼ cup + 1–2 tablespoons low-fat nondairy milk

2–3 tablespoons coconut nectar or pure maple syrup (optional)

In a food processor or high-speed blender (see Note), combine the mango, banana, salt, vanilla, and ¼ cup of the milk. Pulse to get things moving, and then puree, adding the remaining 1 to 2 tablespoons milk if needed. Taste, and add the nectar or syrup, if desired. Serve, or transfer to an airtight container and freeze for an hour or more to set more firmly before serving.

NOTE • If you don't have a high-speed blender, use a food processor instead. While you can use a standard blender here, it has a harder time working through the frozen fruit with this amount of liquid, so you may need more liquid than is optimal for the recipe.

NUTRITIONAL FACTS

Per serving: 116 calories, 1 g protein, 29 g carbohydrates, 22 g sugar, 0.5 g total fat, 4% calories from fat, 2 g fiber, 81 mg sodium

BERRY BUBBLE

MAKES 4 SERVINGS

This spectacular dessert can be made with fresh or frozen berries. Enjoy it any time of year.

Batter Topping

- 1 cup spelt flour
- 2 tablespoons coconut sugar
- 1 teaspoon baking powder
- ½ teaspoon cinnamon
- ⅛ teaspoon sea salt
- ½ cup plain low-fat nondairy milk
- ¼ cup unsweetened applesauce
- 2 teaspoons lemon juice
- 1 teaspoon lemon zest

Berry Base

- 4–4½ cups fresh or frozen berries (see Note)
- 2 tablespoons coconut sugar
- 2 teaspoons tapioca starch
- 1 teaspoon pure vanilla extract
  Pinch of sea salt
- ¼ cup water

Preheat the oven to 350°F.

To prepare the batter topping: In a large bowl, combine the flour, sugar, baking powder, cinnamon, and salt. In a small bowl, combine the milk, applesauce, lemon juice, and lemon zest. Add the wet mixture to the dry and stir until just well combined. The batter should be fairly thick.

To make the fruit base: In an 8" x 8" glass baking dish, combine the berries, sugar, tapioca starch, vanilla, and salt, and toss thoroughly. Add the water and toss again. Roughly distribute the batter over the top of the berry base. (It doesn't need to fully cover the berries.) Bake for about 45 minutes, or until the topping is fully baked through.

NOTE • If using frozen berries, add another 5 to 10 minutes to the baking time.

NUTRITIONAL FACTS
Per serving: 225 calories, 6 g protein, 51 g carbohydrates, 24 g sugar, 1 g total fat, 5% calories from fat, 7 g fiber, 285 mg sodium

CHICKY CHOCOLATE CAKE

MAKES 6 SERVINGS

This cake will surprise you. Don't tell anyone what's in it, just enjoy it! Pair with Magical Chocolate Frosting.

½ cup + 1 tablespoon chickpea flour

½ cup + 1 tablespoon almond meal

¼ cup cocoa powder

1 tablespoon ground chia seeds

1 teaspoon baking soda

⅛ teaspoon sea salt

½ cup aquafaba (the liquid from 1 can of chickpeas or white beans)

⅓ cup + ½–1 tablespoon coconut nectar

1 tablespoon balsamic vinegar

2 teaspoons pure vanilla extract

2 tablespoons nondairy chocolate chips (optional)

Preheat the oven to 350°F. Lightly coat a round cake pan with cooking spray and cover the bottom of the pan with parchment paper.

In a medium bowl, combine the flour, almond meal, cocoa powder, ground chia, baking soda, and salt. Add the aquafaba, nectar, vinegar, and vanilla, and use a whisk to combine well to remove any chickpea flour lumps. Don't worry about overmixing. Add the chocolate chips (if using) and transfer the batter to the prepared cake pan. Bake for about 27 minutes, until a toothpick inserted in the center comes out clean. Transfer the pan to a cooling rack. Let cool completely before removing the cake from the pan.

IDEA: If you want to make this cake into cupcakes, line a muffin pan with 12 parchment cupcake liners, and bake at 350°F for 17 to 18 minutes, or until a toothpick inserted into the center comes out clean.

Shown in color insert pages

NUTRITIONAL FACTS

Per serving: 160 calories, 5 g protein, 23 g carbohydrates, 14 g sugar, 7 g total fat, 36% calories from fat, 4 g fiber, 687 mg sodium

MAGICAL CHOCOLATE FROSTING

MAKES 6 SERVINGS (ENOUGH FROSTING TO COVER A ONE-LAYER CAKE, SUCH AS THE
CHICKY CHOCOLATE CAKE)

This might be the easiest frosting you've ever made, and also the healthiest.

1 cup silken firm tofu or medium-soft tofu, patted dry (see Note)

¼ cup cocoa powder

¼ cup packed pitted dates

½–1 teaspoon pure vanilla extract

½ teaspoon orange or almond extract (if not using full amount of vanilla)

Couple pinches of sea salt

¼–⅓ cup brown rice syrup or thick coconut nectar

In a blender or food processor (not a mixer; it won't smooth the tofu), combine the tofu, cocoa, dates, vanilla extract, orange or almond extract (if using), salt, and ¼ cup of the syrup or nectar. Puree until very smooth. Taste, and add the remaining syrup or nectar to sweeten, if desired. Transfer to a container and refrigerate. (It will thicken more as it cools.)

NOTE • Be sure to use silken here, not standard tofu. They are very different in texture.

Shown in color insert pages

NUTRITIONAL FACTS
Per serving: 94 calories, 4 g protein, 19 g carbohydrates, 8 g sugar, 2 g total fat, 16% calories from fat, 2 g fiber, 122 mg sodium

CHOCOLATE BAKED BANANAS

MAKES 5 SERVINGS

This is one irresistible treat, and you'll be delighted at just how easy it is to prepare!

- 4–5 large ripe bananas, sliced lengthwise
- 2 tablespoons coconut nectar or pure maple syrup
- 1 tablespoon cocoa powder

- Couple pinches sea salt
- 2 tablespoons nondairy chocolate chips (for finishing)
- 1 tablespoon chopped pecans, walnuts, almonds, or pumpkin seeds (for finishing)

Line a baking sheet with parchment paper and preheat oven to 450°F. Place bananas on the parchment. In a bowl, mix the coconut nectar or maple syrup with the cocoa powder and salt. Stir well to fully combine. Drizzle the chocolate mixture over the bananas. Bake for 8 to 10 minutes, until bananas are softened and caramelized. Sprinkle on chocolate chips and nuts, and serve.

IDEA • Serve with a dollop of vanilla nondairy yogurt or a scoop of "nice cream."

Shown in color insert pages

NUTRITIONAL FACTS

Per serving: 146 calories, 2 g protein, 34 g carbohydrate, 18 g sugar, 3 g total fat, 16% calories from fat, 4 g fiber, 119 mg sodium

ACKNOWLEDGMENTS

This book was very much a team effort, and we are very grateful to those who made it happen.

First, thank you to our recipe testers: Carrie Bagnell Horsburgh, Cintia Bock, Sarah Wise, Eve Lynch, Christine Magiera, Michelle Bishop, Natalie Collins, Tami Kramer, Amy Johnson, Don Kearney Bourque, Jenni Mischel, Nina Windhauser, and Kim Davis. Your help and feedback were invaluable. Thank you to Amber Green, RD, for the nutrient analyses. Also thanks to Ashley Flitter for keeping things so well organized and running smoothly. Dreena would like to especially thank Paul, Charlotte, Bridget, and Hope, for sharing her excitement in her work ventures and for keeping it real with recipe feedback.

And a special thank you to Brian DeFiore and Sharon Bowers for your guidance throughout and to Marisa Vigilante for her expert editing and support.

INDEX

An asterisk (*) indicates that photographs appear in the color insert pages.

ABOUT THE AUTHORS

NEAL BARNARD, MD, FACC

Neal Barnard, MD, FACC, is an adjunct associate professor of medicine at the George Washington University School of Medicine in Washington, DC, and president of the Physicians Committee for Responsible Medicine. Dr. Barnard has led numerous research studies investigating the effects of diet on diabetes, body weight, and chronic pain, including a groundbreaking study of dietary interventions in type 2 diabetes, funded by the National Institutes of Health. Dr. Barnard has authored more than 80 scientific publications and 20 books for medical and lay readers. In 2016, he founded the Barnard Medical Center in Washington, DC, as a model for making nutrition a routine part of all medical care.

DREENA BURTON

Dreena Burton is one of the pioneering vegan cookbook authors. Vegan for more than 25 years, Dreena is also a mom to three "weegans." She has charted her journey as a plant-based cook and mother of three through five bestselling cookbooks, including her most recent and beloved title, *Plant-Powered Families.*

Specializing in oil-free whole foods vegan recipes, Dreena's secret ingredient is her passion! Reputed for reliability, her recipes bring whole foods together in unexpected ways to yield delicious flavors and rich textures.

Dreena's recipes are regularly featured by the Physicians Committee for Responsible Medicine, Forks Over Knives, Engine 2 Diet, UC Davis Integrative Medicine, Kris Carr, Blue Zones, The Humane Society, and The Food Network. Connect with Dreena's online community at dreenaburton.com.